JOHN C.

MARY RAC

Foreword by Lee Holden

THE
Five Element
ORCHARD

QiGong Practices for
Harvesting Energy from Trees

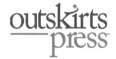

Acknowledgements

We wish to thank and acknowledge the following Masters of Qigong. Their support, teachings, and expertise have helped to shape the concepts and practices in this book.

Master Lee Holden
Dr. Yang, Jwing Ming
Shifu (Cantonese) Jiang Jian-ye
Master Mantak Chia

And a very special thanks and appreciation to Lorelei Chang for her beautiful calligraphy artwork.

DISCLAIMER

The information presented in this book is solely for personal growth, education, and recreation. It is not a therapeutic activity such as psychotherapy, counseling, or medical advice, and it should not be treated as a substitute for any professional assistance or medical care.

Consult with your doctor before beginning this or any other exercise program. In the event of physical or mental distress, please consult with appropriate professionals. Not all exercise programs are suitable for everyone, and this or any other exercise program may result in injury. To reduce the risk of injury, never force or strain. There should never be any be any pain or discomfort during the exercises presented in this book. It any of the movements hurt or are uncomfortable, **stop immediately.** The application of protocols and information in this book is the choice of each practitioner, who assumes full responsibility for his or her understandings, interpretations, and results. The contents of this book are the opinion of its authors, who assume no responsibility for the actions or choices of any practitioner. John and Mary disclaim any liability or loss in connection with the exercises demonstrated by this book.

TABLE OF CONTENTS

FOREWORD

BY LEE HOLDEN

Two Buddhist monks were sitting in the forest in deep meditation. They had been silent for a few hours when one of the monks looks at the other and says, "They call these trees," as he gestures with his arms to the forest. At that point, the two monks burst out in full belly laughter.

What's so comical to the enlightened monks is how we think we know something because we've named it. The mind likes to label and conceptualize. Once we've named something we forget to really look deeper into it. Labeling is the loss of beginners mind. That's why the first passage of the Tao Te Ching says, "The name that can be named is not the real name."

The two monks saw beyond the label, touched the mysterious as they witnessed the trees. They glimpsed the universe through going beyond naming.

Trees are the lungs of the Earth. Nature is your extended body. When you inhale, trees are exhaling. When you exhale, the trees are inhaling. Through practice, we get that visceral sense that everything is connected, that we as humans, are part of an interconnected wholeness.

When we experience this unity, our health and vitality improves, we treat the Earth as a good friend, and develop a harmonious relationship with the world around us.

In this book, John and Mary Platt take us into a practice where we develop a whole new relationship to nature. Not only is this book practical, teaching readers how to boost their life-force energy (Qi) by practicing these techniques, but shows us that we are all part of an interrelated whole.

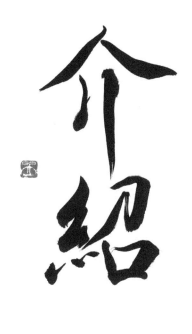

INTRODUCTION

ENERGY FROM TREES

The Magic Red Tree

When I was a young boy, my older brother taunted and captivated me one evening by telling of a magic red tree in the woods outside our house. We lived in an old converted polo pony stable on the edge of several square miles of forest, and the thought of something that special out there was both strange and intoxicating. I was more than fascinated and I planned out ways to find the red tree, but I knew the woods were vast. To me they were just an endless sea of green leaves, briars, and strange noises. I would make little forays out beyond the house, always hoping I would be able to find my way back. The red tree became a holy quest, and I discovered, on each daily journey, that I grew less scared and less worried about getting lost. I discovered that there were mysterious attractions in the woods. The trees became companions, and I began to feel that they spoke to me, comforted and protected me. I could not speak of these things with family members for fear of being branded weird, strange, or crazy. I began to love the woods and I would pass favorite trees and look up into the canopies and watch the sunlight dance in the highest branches. At times, when searching for my magic red tree, I would lie down on the ground and gaze up at the treetops. I would sit with one of the larger trees at my back and feel its presence gently caressing me. I was not alone. I began to understand that there was something in the woods for me, some magical secret, and I was determined to find it. Surely, the red tree would hold the answer. The language of the woods came in the wind through the leaves, the clicking of branches, or the moaning of two trees that rubbed together due to some ice storm or competition for sunlight. But behind it all was a kind of silence, unlike the house noise. I became so at home in this environment of trees and sun and sky that I began to cherish it over home-life and I would practice long periods of silence myself—as if holding onto a secret that no one was to know about. I could not wait each day to go back and continue to look for the magical red tree!

This was my first introduction or induction to the world of trees. From that point on I was enamored, bewitched, and privy to their beauty, both seen and hidden. And the magical red tree? It turned out that my older brother did, in fact, know of a red tree in the forest. I discovered it relatively close to the house where I thought not to look. It was the Christmas tree from the last December whose needles had died and turned red. Yes, it was a red tree, although dead and dull in color. But I did not feel let down, for in the process I had discovered a whole forest of magic.

INTO THE WOODS

There is something silent and magical about the forest. We experience a feeling, a quiet sensibility that settles upon us and allows us to truly see what is around us. We observe the sunlight dancing between the leaves, the scent of pine, the sounds of birds, and stirring animals rustling through the leaves. We have come to a sacred place and we know this because it opens a place inside of us that somehow is the same. We know this place in our deep, quiet times. It is a silent part of us that just observes in stillness. Thus the forest outside becomes an echo of the forest within.

In short, when we enter the woods and walk among trees, we enter another world. We enter a place where we not only feel safe and comfortable, but we also feel healed, refreshed, and rejuvenated. Those giants that we walk among are powerhouses of energy and life-supporting gifts. The benefits of taking a walk in the forest are profuse. But is there a way to tap the energy of trees directly? How do we draw the sweetest nectar of the forest? This book is about techniques, procedures, and ways of connecting. Enter the forest and find your new life.

LEGENDS AND ANCIENT CULTURES

A strong part of my initial fascination with the martial arts, Tai Chi, and internal energy arts was the legends, stories, and exploits of present and past Masters. In the early years of my training, I looked forward to the after class get-togethers and discussions almost as much as I did attending class. Here are just a few:

Martial Arts Master Marshal Yue Fei, who is credited with being the creator of the famous QiGong set called The Eight Pieces of Brocade, was said to have been so fast, so agile, and so powerful in his martial ability, that he quickly advanced to the position of General of the entire Chinese army at the incredibly early age of 25.

I asked one of my Master teachers, "Do you ever get ill?" And his response? "Yes, I get sick on occasion—for about five minutes!"

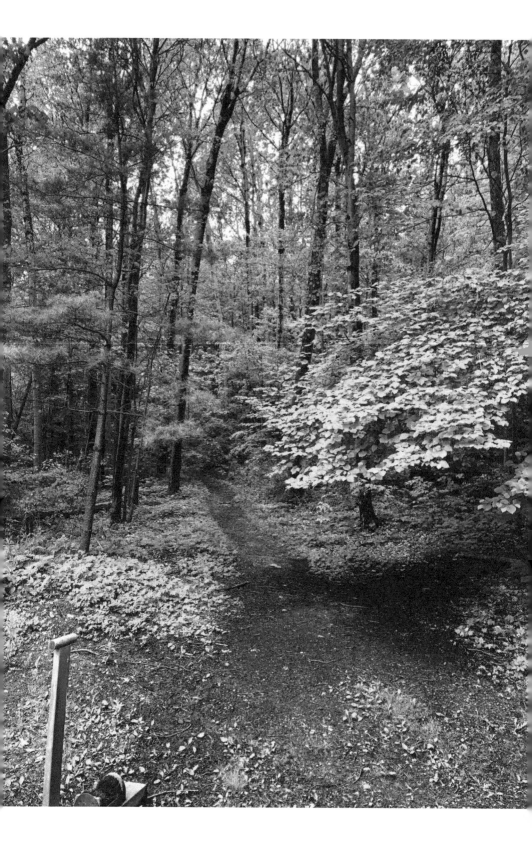

He knew how to energetically work on his own body to avert serious illness.

When we asked our Sifu (teacher) if the legends of Martial Arts Masters having ability to fly through the air was just pure fantasy. His response was, "Well, not entirely."

And what was at the foundation of these and thousands of other legends and stories?

The Vedic Masters of India call it Prana, the Egyptians called it Ra, the Hebrew cabalists called it Ruach, the Native American Lokata Nation call it Wankan; the South Africans call it Ashe, the ancient Romans called it Spiritus. And the ancient and contemporary Taoists called it Qi.

In fact, all cultures with a depth of history and inner development know this subtle, yet wonderfully powerful life-supporting element. Each culture has its legends, techniques, and understandings of what we could call inner energy or that substance that animates life, that energy that runs through all things alive. It propels the planets in their orbits and excites the mitochondria in our cells. It is the light in a young child's face, the sparkle in an old man's eye, the beauty in the sunset, and it is the love in your lover's heart. It flows through channels that the Taoists call meridians and what the Yogis call nadis. It is life itself.

We are born with a finite supply of Qi, yet we have the ability to increase it by absorbing it from the atmosphere, the food we eat, the water we drink, and air that we breathe. To gather and bring in more Qi into the system is to come alive. We gain more energy to circulate through the body, more energy to replace stale or stagnant energy, and more energy to facilitate healing and generate a sense of well-being.

Food, air, and water are our most immediate sources of Qi from the outside. And for most of us, this is what we survive on to keep the body going. But are there other rich sources of energy yet untapped? Did the ancient Taoists know where to go for energy that could do more than just keep us alive? Did they know a secret source?

What the Masters knew was that we all possess this secret energy source. We never lost it. It is always there. However, we cover it with tension, tightness, stress, and a constant flood of thoughts. **We begin to experience Qi energy to the degree to which we let go.** The Masters have been writing about and teaching ways to let go and relax for centuries. Both mind and body begin to settle down, and we learn to live in present moment awareness.

A simple story of two fish makes this point: Two fish were swimming along and enjoying the morning. A third fish swam by and said, "Hi guys, how's the water today?" and swam on. After a few moments, one fish looked at the other and said, "Do you have any idea what he is talking about? What is water?"

ENERGY FROM THE SUN

We are light driven beings, and, as such, the sun is a tremendous source of energy. In fact, it is our primary source of energy. In India the spiritual teachers tells us that the Sun God is nature's best healer. Life on earth exists because of sunlight.

We are light driven beings

Light is energy, and it is in our best interest to cultivate it. Light could also be called a type of electromagnetic radiation that is composed of a combination of particles and wave function. This is why it can move so fast and can move through a vacuum. We take light into our bodies through breathing and the food we eat. Plants are stored sunlight. They transfer sunlight through the process of photosynthesis. We are eating stored sunlight! We could say, then, that our bodies are "light driven." The medical profession has long recognized

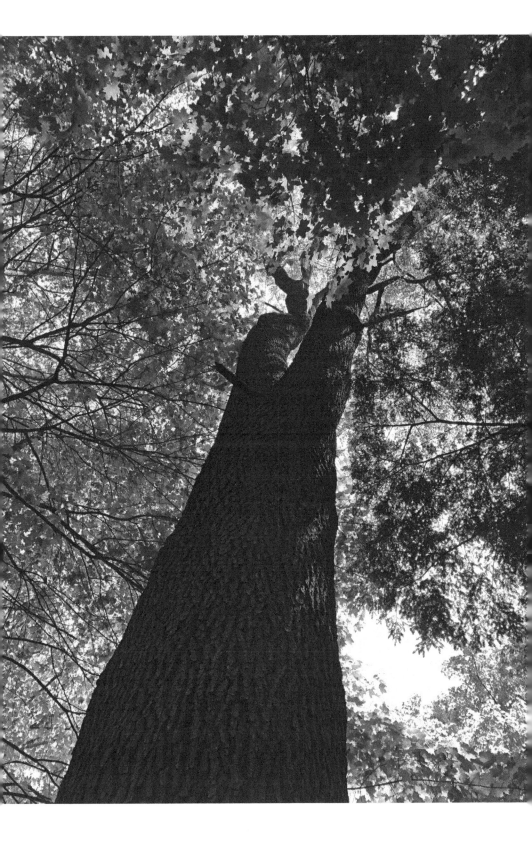

that a lack of sunlight (especially in the winter season) can produce "seasonal disorder." The early Qigong masters discovered that we can infuse light into an organ to change negative emotions to positive. The use of a specific color on a particular organ can bring about transformations.

TREE QI

This energy source that we call Qi, Prana, Ka, Ki, etc., is alive in all things living and non-living. In Japan there is a growing tradition called Shinrin Yoku, which means "Forest Bathing." Daily buses leave the city of Tokyo bringing hundreds of people to the forest in search of the healing that the forest can provide. The Taoist Masters have long prescribed a simple action for well-being and even healing—"breathe the air of trees!" It is difficult to walk in the forest for a period of time and not come out feeling refreshed, rejuvenated and cleansed. On one such walk, one of my teachers asked if we wanted to learn how to see the human aura. Naturally attracted to all things esoteric, I immediately said, "Yes." He then explained that it is best to start with trees, as their auras are stronger, bigger, and easier to recognize. And so we stood silently looking at the crown of the canopy of a large, prominent pine tree in the distance. The glow that was around the tree was unmistakable—bright and strong. I began to look at the auras of other trees, each one having a distinct "halo." It was separate from the canopy, yet still very much a part of it. "When you become good at tree aura recognition, it is an easy step to human auras," the teacher explained. But before the end of the forest walk, I realized something very special. These energy extensions of trees were not limited to the top of the canopy. In fact, I realized that the energy emanated from these forest giants in all directions, at any level. I was walking through auras! When we walk through the forest, we are moving through and breathing in an interconnecting "mesh" of multiple auras. Was this the true meaning of the term, "Forest

Bathing?" Would walking through a pine forest be a different "bath" than walking through an apple orchard?

These forest bathing experiences were my first entry into the power, the energy, and wonderful beauty of Tree energy or the Qi of Trees. The common tree is a super rich source of energy. And this book provides the serious practitioner with methods to tap this incredible energy source. And trees are happy to give it!

"The contemplation of nature can free you of that 'me,' the great trouble maker." Eckhart Tolle (3)

"Nature {Trees} can bring you to stillness. That is its gift to you. When you perceive and join with nature in the field of stillness, that field becomes permeated with your awareness." Eckhart Tolle (4)

This book will cover multiple approaches to absorbing energy from trees. Each approach has a number of variations and pathways to do this. In the final chapter the reader is invited to put together their own combination of techniques. Here then is a series of methods to absorb Qi from trees that you can put into your "toolbox" to use any time that you're outside in the forest, park, or backyard.

Chapter Overview

Chapter 1 Metaphor

This chapter outlines the tree as a metaphor for how inner energy works in the human body. It explains how the tree's canopy, trunk, and roots all mirror the three basic categories of Internal Energy: Heaven, Mankind, and Earth Energies. The metaphor will become the template for all the other chapters as well as the main thesis.

- Learn how trees have a wisdom that, in some ways, we have lost.
- Learn what we share with these giants of energy, silent power, and patience.

Chapter 2 Connecting to Nature

Here the reader is introduced to how one can tap into and use the three forces of nature mentioned in Chapter 1. This chapter starts with an explanation of how and why we have moved away from nature, as well as our ability to re-connect to natural forces outside the body. The chapter then moves into ways to connect: rooting, protecting, and relaxing. Starting in this chapter, you will learn specific techniques to connect with, and gather, energy from trees.

- Reconnect using Nature.
- Learn grounding, centering, and balancing from the Masters—the Trees!

Chapter 3 How to approach a Tree

This short chapter introduces the idea that a tree is a living, feeling entity. Readers learn how to choose and approach a tree for energy absorption. Finding the right tree is often done with intuition and feeling.

- Learn the silent language of the forest.
- Learn to let the healing tree find you.

Chapter 4 Absorbing Tree Energy

With the foundation of the three sources of energy and the tree as metaphor for these forces, the reader is introduced to different standing poses to do while near the tree chosen for practice. Each stance allows the body to absorb energy from the tree in a different way, bringing tree energy into a different part of the body, or for a specific healing purpose.

- Learn how to stand correctly to absorb energy into a particular organ or area of the body for healing.
- Learn how to line up your meridian lines to allow a free flow of energy from within and from without.
- Learn a special technique using "Octopus" hands to absorb energy from trees directly.

Chapter 5 Follow the Sun

Trees seek nourishment from earth and the atmosphere, and most importantly the sun. Learning how a tree grows and where the strongest energy in a tree is at any given times of the day gives us knowledge of how to choose from what side of the tree to seek energy, as well as the understanding of the best times to practice tree energy absorption.

- Learn how the sun is perhaps the most important element in tree energy practice.
- Learn how to know where to stand next to a tree to get the most energy.

Chapter 6 The Five Element Orchard

The reader is first introduced to the Chinese Five Element Theory. The reader will begin to understand that different kinds of trees have different effects on specific organs or diseases.

- Learn how to use the odors of a tree as potent medicine.
- Learn how to use the tree's color to harmonize your own system.
- Learn what the ancient Masters knew about specific trees for specific healing needs.
- Learn which trees you have in the back yard or park that are best for you.

Chapter 7 Orbits of Energy

Energy is continually circulating in both trees and humans. This chapter shows us how to tap into the energy orbits of trees and blend this power with our own, creating a tree/human orbit of energy.

- Learn to circulate tree energy into your own system.
- Learn to mix your energy with that of your chosen tree.

Chapter 8 Life Blood of the Tree

In this chapter participants are given the directions to actually move and feel the energy of trees. This is an extremely powerful practice, and it gives us a profound understanding of our own internal energy.

- Learn how to move tree energy.

Chapter 9 Putting it all Together

As described in the previous chapters, there are numerous ways to harvest energy from trees. In this section the reader is given various ways to put these techniques together to make a practice that is most enjoyable and rewarding. This will help you to develop your own personal practice, so when you next visit the forest, you are prepared with a "toolbox" of techniques.

Chapter 10 Fields Beyond the Orchard

This final chapter takes us beyond the Five Elements and tree energy practice. Here are a number of nature and forest exercises that can be wonderful additions to your practice as you venture outside. Each exercise is unique and intended to bring you yet closer to nature, closest to your true self. Enjoy them!

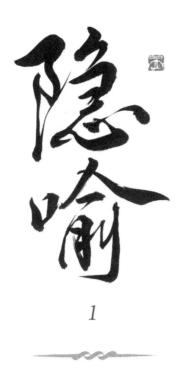

1

METAPHOR

Roughly 4500 years ago, something astounding was introduced to Chinese culture. The now classic text of Chinese philosophy, the *Yi Jing,* first expressed the concept that natural energy or power was of three kinds: Heaven energy, Earth energy, and Man's own internal energy. These were called San Cai (the three primordial, natural sources of energy). All three forces were subject to cycles and natural law; thus man was seen as intimately connected to the other two forces and subject to nature's cycles. This idea was to become one of the basic tenets of the Chinese philosophy of Taoism.

Some historians believe that learning about the relationship and interaction of these three forces was the start of that practice known as Qigong—defined as the effort and time used to study Qi or energy in the human body.

With the understanding of mankind's relationship with both

heaven and earth energy, the early Masters began to see the human body as a conduit between the two, and that we actually had access to two unbounded energy sources. They also came to understand that if we could purify our energy enough, it could match the energy of heaven, which they believed was more pure, of higher quality, and of a higher vibration. Matching our energy to heaven energy was a way of forming a greater connection to the universe, a spiritual bond. The idea was to tune the violin of the self to the orchestra of nature.

On a deep intuitive level we know that we have a primordial connection to heaven and earth energies. Consider the common phrases: "Reach for the stars," "I'm in heaven," "I live here, but my roots are in the highlands," "I feel grounded," "My spirit soars." Qigong Masters have developed such sensitivity and awareness that these become more than euphemisms. They have learned to actually feel their connection to the cosmos and to the earth.

In the 1960's Western scientists began investigating the concept of internal energy, something that almost all ancient cultures know intimately. The ethereal nature of Qi was a difficult hurdle, but just as we can feel wind on the face without seeing it, Qi could be experienced in terms of outcome, results, and feeling. In an effort to maintain a respectable scientific objectivity, Western scientists labeled it as "Bio-electromagnetic" energy. "Electro" being that aspect of energy that spans our atmosphere and beyond. Magnetic is a referral to earth's magnetic pull and consequential energy power. Bio, of course, is the energy in the human body, which animates us, keeps our organs working, pumps our blood, and basically runs the whole metabolic process that we call life. But here for the first time the Western scientific mind was beginning to comprehend the concept of forces inside the human body that were, in fact, an integral part of its functioning. The concept of the three forces, called "San Cai," is bioelectric magnetic energy—East meets West!

Early Taoist cosmology states that from the primordial force (The Tao) came two—yin and yang. The *Tao Te Ching* says, "One gave birth to two," and these two forces became polarities, which govern the cycles, movement, and direction of the entire universe—light and dark, life and death, male and female. Yin and Yang were not seen as two different types of energy but simply the complementary poles of opposites upon which life functions. The early Chinese Masters characterized the energy of the heavens as being positively charged, expansive, and outwardly flowing. This heaven energy was considered more of a Yang energy—electric and full of power. The earth energy was seen as Yin: inward flowing, receptive and negatively charged—magnetic. However, when it comes to the human body, we need to understand that it truly is a conduit between these two heaven and earth forces. And like all things in nature, the human form constantly seeks balance. In fact, Qigong could be described as those procedures (movement, breathing, and mental attention), which allow the Yin and Yang polarities in our body to balance and even out. Traditional Chinese Medical doctors tell us that almost all illness can be traced to an imbalanced yin and yang. The first way to initiate this balance is to allow the Qi or life energy in our bodies to move and circulate freely, eliminating areas of stagnation, constriction, or tightness.

These early medical doctors knew that when energy does not flow freely through its channels, called meridians, the body's energy will stagnate. It is much like a boulder rolling down onto a stream and causing one side of the stream to flood and stand still, and the other side to become arid and dry. In reality, stagnation is often caused by constriction, brought about by poor posture, too much sitting, or lack of movement. Another area of stagnation could be caused by pollution from the food, water, and air quality that we ingest. This would also include emotional pollution—our worries, fears, angers, and anxieties. Perhaps the greatest cause for energy stagnation in our modern society is tightness in the body caused by stress. We often don't realize that stress can cause us to recoil and momentarily go into a state that has been called, "fight or flight." This is needed at times, but when the nervous system is constantly exposed to stressful situations, it is the body that receives the damage in the form of tightness. We tense up to prepare for the fight or the flight, but this tightness stays with us long after the stressful event, and the Qi flow is hampered.

When this stagnation reaches the point where there is organ failure, problematic symptoms or lasting pain, the Traditional Chinese doctor will incorporate acupuncture, herbs, and massage techniques to remove the stagnant areas and get the energy flowing again. In terms of prevention and strong energy, the layman has great recourse in the movement and breathing patterns of Qigong.

In addition to the techniques of traditional Qigong exercise programs, the practitioner is always advised to ingest pure food, water, and clean air when possible. The Masters have long known the benefits of taking an active role in maintaining one's health and well being. There is something potent in those health activities that one engages in. Here you take an active role; whereas, the Western approach is to take medicine or have a procedure performed—a passive approach.

And they found that example in abundance: the tree, the perfect metaphor.

To this end the Masters needed a model, a pure example of energy, balanced Yin and Yang. They needed another entity, other than human, that acted like a conduit between heaven and earth, one that could actually give energy, strength, and healing properties. They needed a perfect example of the vast energy field of nature. And they found that example in abundance in the tree, the perfect metaphor.

The tree's canopy rises up and reaches for the sun, gathering energy, light, and strength. It is the Yang of the tree, that part that expands, stretches, and charges. Through photosynthesis, the light of the sun, the tree is charged with energy, allowing the tree to give off oxygen, life-giving negative ions, and its special odor.

Tree roots sink deep into the earth, gathering, processing, and using earth's nutrients and powerful magnetic energy. This is the Yin of the tree—inward, passive, accepting. A popular type of green tea called Pu-erh only grows in the Provence of Yunnan China, where the soil, altitude, and ecosystem allows this special tea to charge with its wonderful properties. It is said that the small tree or bush of the Pu'erh has roots that extend down four times its height. With this much emphasis on earth energy for growth, Pu-erh has often been called the "Tea of Qi."

> When we walk through a forest setting, we are actually walking through a complex web of ethereal energy…

On a more spiritual level, trees produce and maintain magnificent auras that extend well beyond the trunk, branches, and canopy. When we walk through a forest setting, we are actually walking through a complex web of ethereal energy produced by trees that cross, mix, and blend. All this is accomplished with the greatest stillness and patience. Trees are still, all the time watching and remembering. It is their dharma, their allotted duty on earth.

What can we learn from this abundant, ever-present, and one of nature's most perfect examples of primordial forces at work? Trees reach for the sun, and as such, become one with and connected to the air, sky, and cosmos. Yet they sink deep into the earth, becoming rooted, centered, and connected, as well.

When the *Yi Ching* expounded on the idea that mankind is intimately connected to three forces, as are trees, it was a way to see our connection to nature. If we could match our energy to the energy of the heavens, might we live longer and enjoy greater health and mental balance? If we could root our energy into the earth, might we become more centered?

> …powerful dynamos of life giving energy that we can gather from, exchange with, and purify.

The tree becomes our metaphor for understanding how three forces work together and harmonize. But the greatest gift the trees have for us is that they are powerful dynamos of life giving energy from which we can gather and exchange.

This short book is a series of Qigong practices that are designed to use energy from trees. These techniques and procedures come from several of the greatest living Qigong Masters of our time. Through ancient teaching practices and knowledge of how internal energy works in both mankind and in trees, these Masters have given us an incredibly rich resource. With our metaphor of the human body as a tree, we can begin to understand that the comparison is really one of inner energy and how that energy works and moves in the body. We have much to learn from trees.

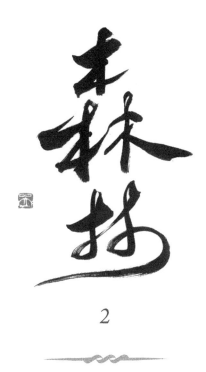

2

CONNECTING TO NATURE

How we long to achieve the growth the tree fosters in itself, the reach and rootage, the sturdiness and balance between high and low, the way it meets each season, holding its ground, space or blooming. (1)

We stand rooted to the forces of earth, and with this grounding we feel centered, steady, and secure. We feel a "heavenly pull," as if a golden thread is pulling up the crown of the head. We feel proud, balanced, and courageous. Our arms move up the body overhead and spread to the sides, fingers wide like leaves of a giant oak, absorbing sunlight.

The first step in absorbing energy from trees is to build on the idea of the tree as a metaphor and learn how to connect to nature. We learn what trees have always known—the necessity to sink roots deep into the earth, how to keep a strong, protective covering, and how to be silent and rest in the present moment. In Peter Wohlleben's book, *The Hidden Life of Trees,* we learn that trees care and feed one another. They have intricate social systems and sophisticated language systems. In short, we can learn much about how our own system of inner energy works by observing nature. The Taoists have been doing this for thousands of years. And there is no better start than to learn from trees—learn the benefits of making a strong connection to earth, the environment, and the cosmos. Learn how to stretch the body to dilate meridian lines and remove energy stagnation from muscles and tendons. And perhaps most importantly, learn how to relax and flow with life's currents.

To connect and learn from trees is a profound, concrete way of making a reconnection with nature. In fact, we begin to learn how to connect to the whole cosmos, a practice the ancient Taoists thought was so important to our well-being.

When did we loose our connection to nature? At what point did modern life create problems greater than the ones it was solving? Towards the end of the nineteenth and beginning of the twentieth centuries, three significant things began to happen. Although the industrial age had been part of European and American life for some decades at that point, we now began to become a working industrial nation. We began to live by the clock, not by the sun. In ever increasing numbers, we began to work in factories, not in fields. And we began to feel less connected, more fragmented. Secondly, we began to move off the farms into cities in huge numbers. We became a country of large metropolises, no longer a country of small farms, almost overnight. We started to lose touch with the earth, that for centuries had been our source of work, food, and social base. The third major event of the time period was the utter devastation of the First World War. For the first time we experienced a war involving major countries and weapons of mass destruction. These events prompted a new worldview and way of looking at ourselves that was totally different. We became more alienated from one another, fragmented and ungrounded.

The Power of Rooting

Our modern harried life has produced untold problems, both mental and physical. And perhaps the greatest assault upon our bodies and souls comes from what we have moved away from, increasingly over the years. And what is that one thing? Nature. We watch screens, not sunsets. We walk on sideways in asphalt jungles, instead of on wooded paths in the forest. We breath the air filled with carbons, we don't breathe the air of trees.

Because we lost our connection with Mother Earth, we no longer feel grounded, stable, or at ease. The Taoists have long known the value of feeling connected to earth, and it has been an important part of any energy practice. Without this connection there is no root, no balance. When Qigong entered its martial phase, in or near the Song dynasty in roughly 600 A.D., the warriors began to realize the value and power of using internal energy to connect and root to earth, making them stronger in battle, better able to defend, better able to deliver a strike against the enemy. However, the early Taoists had known centuries before that a strong connection to earth meant a connection of the soul, a connection to that which nourishes us and provides our needs. That connection meant health and longevity.

To attack one who is rooted, is to attempt to attack earth itself.

Rooting means to form a firm mental and physical connection to earth beyond just standing on it or feeling the weight of gravity. For the martial artist it meant establishing a base from which to defend and attack. However, rooting can mean far more. Rooting to earth forms our platform from which we see and operate in this world. If we are firmly rooted to the earth like a tree when we encounter physical, mental, emotional, or even psychic attacks, we have a strong ally. To attack one who is rooted is to attack earth itself. And she can take it! In fact, Qigong Masters often talk about sending our negativity, our stagnant energy, or our emotional turmoil back down to earth, where it will be recycled, so to speak. As Master Lee Holden says, "Let Mother Earth take your negativity. She will use it as compost."

Conversely, we live in a world where we are almost constantly being uprooted. We speak of it as loosing our center, not feeling grounded, or feeling unsettled. Nothing does this faster than the stress many of us have to experience daily. Stress often translates in the body as tightness, especially in the shoulder and neck region, but also in other places. This pulls us away from our feeling of being settled or grounded. To reconnect to the forces of earth is to mitigate the effects of stress.

So, our first step in connecting to trees is to learn how to root. Simple!

The following techniques are ways to connect. Some of them involve a strong sense of imagery and others are more visceral or physically oriented. However, they all involve your focused attention. Remember the importance of using your attention to direct the Qi. Here we simply use it to connect our energy with earth energy.

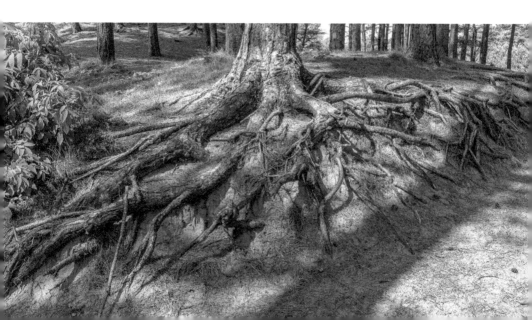

Wuji

Wuji is the state of no extremity, no discrimination. It is a state of nothingness. According to Taoist cosmology, at the beginning of the universe there was no limit or measurement—just emptiness. It becomes a metaphor for the mind. Wuji is the neutral state, without emotions or desires. Buddhists use the term "no mind." In this state Qi is not led away, thus you can conserve and build it.

The Wuji standing posture borrows from this concept and calls for a stance of complete stillness. It is the body's equivalent of mental transcendence.

In practice one stands in a posture that aligns the major energy lines in the body so as not to impede the flow. The stillness allows energy to run through its channels unimpeded without angles or congestion.

Getting to Wuji

1. Stand comfortably with the feet shoulder width apart. Let your arms hang comfortably at your sides. Be attentive to nine points at the bottom of the feet: the five toes, two balls of the foot, the center of the foot and the heel, making sure your weight is evenly distributed on these nine points. Check for even weight distribution and a feeling of evenness.

2. Create a slight crease at the ankle level of both feet, keeping the feet and ankles soft, even, and steady.

3. Next, bring awareness to the knees and make them "soft." There should only be a slight bend at the knees.

4. Let your awareness come up to the sacrum below the small of your back. Gently tuck the sacrum in. How far to tilt may involve some experimentation as you would adjust the rabbit ears on an early model TV set. Adjust the tilt until you feel the energy transference from the feet into the body.

5. Mentally come up to your back between the two shoulder

blades. Gently spread or separate these outward and, at the same time, slightly round the shoulders, allowing your arms to hang down at your sides. You will also feel a slight space in your arms pits with this action.

6. Next, pull the chin in slightly, allowing your crown to face straight up toward the sky. Once your body is aligned in this way, keep the structure, but relax.

The Wuji stance is an important step in rooting the body to earth. If the body is settled, balanced, and at ease, one easily finds a comfortable relationship with gravity and begins to feel grounded.

Wuji Stance

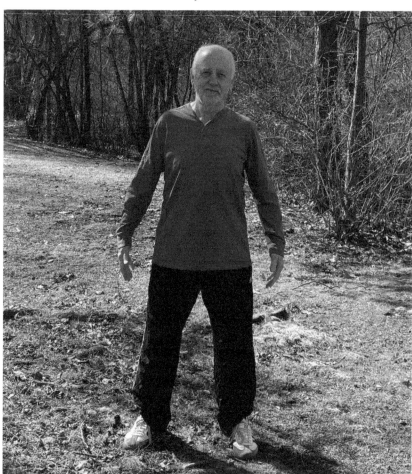

Benefits of the Wuji Stance

This stance will be used with many of the techniques in this book, especially with the various standing postures in Chapter Three. From Wuji the whole universe unfolds. From the Wuji stance, we can move into a wide variety of poses that allow us to directly receive energy from trees. This stance is truly a "standing meditation," as the body achieves an effortless stillness. And in this physical stillness, we essentially line up the energy lines or meridians in the body and we begin to experience the flow of energy surging through the body. Often people experience energy in the body for the first time in this simple standing posture.

DEVELOPING "TREE ROOTS"

Our forest friends, the trees, not only sink deep into the earth, but their roots also form a way to communicate and actually help other trees of like-species. Trees receive nourishment from Mother Earth and, at the same time, have protection against the harshness of the elements. To have deep roots is to have both connection and protection.

> **Procedure**. Stand in Wuji stance for a few minutes and let the body settle down. Feel a stronger sense that you are not only standing on a huge ball, but that you are part of it.

Imagine and feel as if you have roots coming from the bottom of your feet and sinking into the earth. Feel this root structure extend down from the bottom of your feet for four, six, even nine feet into the earth. The relaxed meridian lines that carry our internal energies, as a result of standing in the Wuji stance will allow you to feel the earth energy. With practice you will actually feel the magnetic earth energy coming up into the body, the same way earth nutrients come into the tree.

Benefits. With extended practice this feeling of your imaginary roots sinking into the earth with the Wuji stance will give you a much greater sense of being grounded, balanced, and centered. You will develop your earth connection and have an ally against invasion of any kind, be it pathogenic or psychic. Your emotions will settle down, and stress will slowly leave your body and descend to earth.

Tree Roots II

Tai Chi Master and author John Loupos takes this rooting concept one step deeper. He shows us how to root using the whole lower half of the body, not just from the bottoms of the feet.

Procedure. Stand in Wuji stance as before, but this time imagine that you're in the earth up to your waist. Imagine you are a large plant with your upper body and head as the leaves and flowers. Imagine that your two legs are two of many roots that extend deep into the earth, four to nine feet deep.

Benefits. This rooting from the waist should give you an even greater sense of connection. The whole body will feel extremely anchored and your ability to imagine and feel earth's power will be even greater. Nothing can move you!

Strengthening the Core and the Guardian Qi

Continuing the concept of the Tree as metaphor for understanding our relationship with heaven, earth, and our own forces, we move to the trunk. It is the foundation, which supports the root system, limbs, and canopy.

THE HORSE STANCE—STRENGTHENING THE BELT CHANNEL

There is a legend of how the horse stance became an important martial arts standing position. In the southern part of China in cities near large rivers or ocean, whole families were born, grew up and worked on the large Chinese boats called junks. Currents and tides would continually rock these vessels, and this was one of the few places people had to train in martial arts, either because of circumstance or secrecy. Because of the continuous rocking, practitioners adopted what was to become the Horse Stance—a low, wide-leg squatting position, as if riding a horse. This would give them stability and a power base from which to defend and strike. Whether the legend is true or not, this stance does, in fact, afford the practitioner much more than stability. There are numerous advantages to this position, but the greatest benefit, perhaps, is the way that the practitioner can feel connected to their center and core or belt channel.

In the late 1960's when I was quite young and an ardent practitioner of the martial arts, I trained with Sifu Al Dacascos (now Grandmaster). One night he had his students get into the horse stance. Little did we suspect he was to leave us in this stance for 40 minutes. Protocol, respect, and honor prohibited any one of us to even think about coming out of the stance, despite intense pain, heat, and heavy breathing. When released from the pose, we felt tired, full of aches and pain. We assumed, of course, that we had endured this challenge to demonstrate endurance and discipline, as well as strengthen the leg muscles.

Many years later that I learned that this very stance also gave me a way to develop and strengthen the internal Qi channel called the belt or girdle vessel. Without this horizontal channel at the waist level, we would lose all sense of equilibrium and balance.

Secondly, and perhaps more importantly, the horse stance lowers the perineum or pelvic floor to the earth, thus reinforcing our natural, but lost, connection to the ground.

Procedure. First stand in Wuji stance and feel yourself begin to settle down to the earth. Allow your muscles to hang off your bones like clothes hanging on a coat hanger. Next separate your feet so that they are approximately three feet apart. Keeping your spine straight, begin to lower your body by slowly bending your knees. Be sure to keep your toes pointed straight ahead and apply outward pressure on your knees, aligning your knees directly over your ankles. (Caution—this pose can be quite problematic for those with weak knees or lack of experience with bending the knees down. Avoid this exercise if you feel discomfort or pain directly in the knees.) Once in a fairly low, almost squatting position, place your hands on your hips, while placing your mind on the perineum (located between the anus and the genitals). Feel the connection to the earth. Feel the earth energy enter this area of the body. You can also start to feel this earth connection in the bottoms of the feet. Stand in this position for 1 or 2 minutes. Come out slowly.

Benefits. Lowering the perineum closer to the ground will allow earth energy to respond and bounce back. Your belt channel will strengthen, and this will greatly enhance your protective layer of Qi energy that surrounds your body called Wei Qi. This in turn will improve your immune functioning. Your ability to resist pathogens will improve. The longer you are able to stay in the stance, the more you will start to feel a tremendous sense of strength and power.

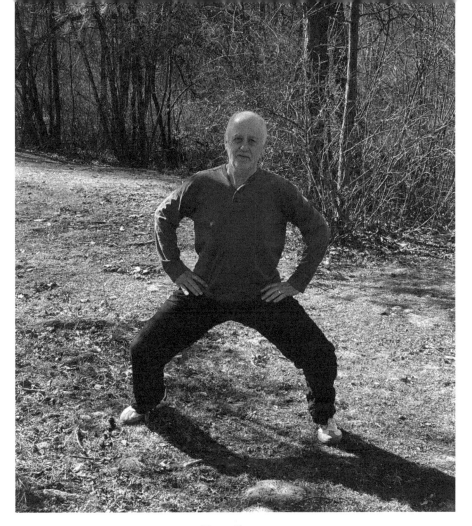

Horse Stance

ABDOMINAL BREATHING

When more and more Qigong masters began to bring these ancient energy techniques to America, they were surprised to note how much we sat and how shallow our breathing was in general. Abdominal Breathing is one of those Qigong techniques that is simple, yet beneficial in so many ways. It allows us to bring in much greater amounts of oxygen and Qi, which, in turn, has benefits for the entire system. It is an excellent way to strengthen our core, our storehouse of energy.

Procedure. This simple breathing technique can be done either in a standing or sitting position. Place both your hands one over the other at your abdomen, just below your belly button. As you inhale, allow the air to come in and expand your abdomen. In actuality the air can go no further than the diaphragm, yet the Qi is not restricted by these boundaries. Upon inhaling, the abdomen expands out, and as you exhale you gently push the abdomen back towards the spine. Repeat this process as long as you feel comfortable. Your breath should be long, slow, deep, and soft.

Benefits. The benefits from this breathing technique are many. Here are just a few: As you breathe in and push the diaphragm down, you are gently massaging the internal organs. Sitting or standing hunched over has the tendency to constrict these organs preventing a free flow of energy. When you breathe into the lower lobes of the lungs, nerve endings are activated triggering the parasympathetic nervous system (often called the "relaxation response"). As the diaphragm pushes down, it not only massages the organs, but also pushes gently on the adrenal and pancreas glands, allowing a release of hormones needed for better metabolism. All these actions create an antidote to stress. Do this breathing often and for as long as is comfortable. It is a great way to stay calm behind the wheel of your car (both hands on the steering wheel, of course). Perhaps the greatest benefit of Abdominal Breathing is its ability to strengthen what is called "The Elixir Field" below the navel and the Guardian Qi (energy that surrounds the body) at the same time.

QI BELT BREATHING

Qi Belt Breathing directly affects the Guardian Qi by allowing the breath and your attention to go outwards towards the skin. This strengthens the energy around the mid-section, which, in turn, affects the whole body. The early Taoist practitioners looked for ways to make the body impervious to disease. The idea was to develop and practice those procedures that put a protective coat around you. In later centuries, the martial artists were to use this concept to make soldiers more resilient to attack.

Procedure. Hold the hands at waist level. Form a "claw" with your first finger and thumb wide on each side, leaving the

Qi Belt Breathing

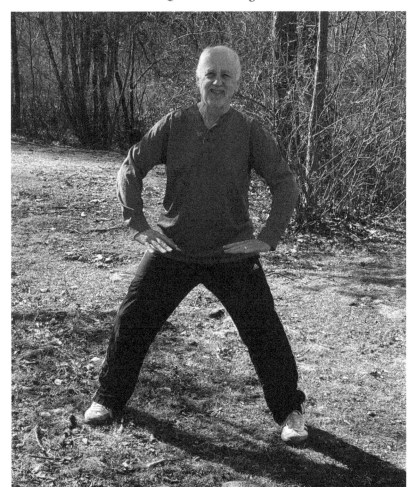

remaining fingers free. Inhale deeply and draw your attention and breathe to the inside of the mid-section. Exhale and let the sides of your lungs and mid-section expand outward. Let your mind lead the Qi both inward and outward. Repeat this breathing for 36 times.

Benefits. This kind of breathing with attention directs your energy. Here the benefit is for your skin and its protective covering. This will build your immune system, your Guardian Qi.

Additional Ways to build the Guardian Qi

Because of the importance of having this strong covering, Qigong Masters developed many ways to strengthen the Guardian Qi. Here are a few additional ways:

- A daily professional or self massage
- Light knocking or slapping on the whole body
- Qigong exercises for blood and Qi circulation

RELAXATION

Often taught as the first and most important element in internal energy practices such as Tai Chi, Qigong and Yoga, is the practice of relaxing or letting go. We will feel the energy during these practices to the extent to which we can let go and relax the system.

When we think of relaxing, we think of letting go, becoming "loose," releasing tension, not caring. Qigong Masters, in fact, often talk about layers of relaxation, from relaxing the musculature to actually learning how to relax the internal organs! One of the most important reasons to relax is that the reduction of tension on the body allows the meridian lines through which Qi or internal energy flows to dilate. Tight muscles will close the lines and the flow will diminish or stop. This is a major difference between Eastern and Western exercise methods. Can we learn to relax while we move? The results of doing this are profound!

To be like a tree is to relax and just be. It does not include extra effort or intense practice. The tree just stands, it just is. When we learn this skill, we learn the secret to life, longevity, and radiant health. Two concepts that speak so well to this philosophy come from Japan and China: The Japanese practice of Forest Bathing and Taoist teaching of non-action.

Although I had been practicing martial arts, along with long periods of daily meditation, I really had no experience of complete relaxation until I happened to be on a meditation retreat in Massachusetts about 30 years ago. One day in meditation I was feeling particularly tired and decided to simply lie down, just breathe and take it easy for a while. My skin started to feel a little warm, and I just put my attention on the outer layer of my body as if I were wrapping myself in a blanket of awareness. All of a sudden my body turned into a furnace of brilliant light, and I felt an electric, buzzing sensation throughout. I had no idea what was happening, but the experience was blissful. I must have stayed in this flood of light and feeling for over an hour, because friends came in to tell me I was about to miss dinner! Needless to say, the practice of lying down after meditation became a recurring part of my daily practice from that point on.

It was not until about 12 years later when I started studying Qigong with Master Ron Diana in New Jersey that I came to understand my on-going experience. Ron was teaching Mantak Chia's technique of Micrcocosmic Orbit meditation. This was a different kind of meditation for me, and it involved more imagery and feeling the energy as it looped through my body. At one point Ron stated that, with practice, one could experience a blissful feeling of Qi throughout the body as the energy circulated. So that was what I was experiencing—Qi!! This then became my first awakening to how energy in the body feels, as well as the tremendous effect it had on my mind. I began to realize that the gate, or trigger to this blissful feeling of energy was something ever so simple—relaxation. Learning to relax opened the floodgates of Qi. With more experience, training, and the help of more great teachers, I learned that through relaxation, attention, and a little technique I could heal my body, and increase my mental faculties. This was the magic ingredient of the Taoist alchemist. Relaxation was essential—to transform lethargy to strong physical energy, negative emotions to positive, and mental worries to wisdom.

FOREST BATHING

One practice that uses nature to emphasize relaxation is called "Forest Bathing." In Japan there is a growing number of people who have adopted the practice of "Shinrin Yoko," or "Forest Bathing." Each day hundreds of enthusiasts get on a bus that takes them to forested areas. Their strong belief is that nature and the green landscape of trees, vegetation, and whole forests can heal us, simply by our being in it—bathing. There has been much written about the power of "getting back to nature." Just as we have lost our rooting and our ability to feel grounded, we have left nature for unnatural environments. Shinrin Yoko practitioners have abundant techniques and practices, which allow them to get in touch with and get back to natural forces. Many of these activities include observing nature's own relaxation. This, in turn, brings them into the present moment—a much more relaxing place to be. One such practice is simply to observe the movement of nature. Participants are asked to continue gazing at some part of the natural environment that gently moves. This could be long grass gently swaying in a field, or the floating movement of aspen leaves. This continuous observation, researchers claim, begins to change the brain chemistry and the body starts to relax and settle.

Forest Bathing

Procedure. Find a pleasant wooded trail that, preferably, goes in a loop of a mile or less. The forested area should contain a diverse ecosystem with a mix of conifers. If your trail passes a pond, stream, river or ocean, it is even better. Just walk and enjoy the scenery. Walk in silence and breathe deeply—settle into the present moment. "Breathe the air of trees." Use all your senses to deepen your experience. Listen to the wind in the trees, watch the subtle, rhythmic motion of the treetops, and feel the intersecting webs of tree auras.

WU WEI

The Chinese word, "Wu Wei" is often translated as "non-doing." More accurately, it means the very least amount of action—action that does not require extra effort or work. This is a Taoist concept that emphasizes being natural, not over—doing. In this way you act with the direction of the natural flow of nature—the Tao.

Although there are numerous ways to explain this practice along with numerous examples, it basically means to "do just enough." Over exertion or too much of anything has its price. Just do what is required and then relax. Perhaps the phrase that best demonstrates this Taoist approach of non-action is "do less and accomplish more." The very idea of relaxing and just letting things happen is often considered too foreign, too passive for us in our busy world of more and more. We persist in the notion that to relax is to weaken and negate accomplishment. The idea of working just enough and relaxing often presupposes that we will fail. But the Taoists say that there are natural forces at work; more specifically, the force of nature, the Tao, is in charge of all movement and you need only go with the flow of life—all will get done. It is a strange concept to the Western thinker, but it forms the very center of Tai Chi movement and philosophy.

In nature, nothing is in excess, overdone, or effort oriented. Nature is Wu Wei perfected. If we are to "tune the violin of the self to the orchestra of nature," we will have to adopt an attitude and practice of economy. In short, we just need to relax and allow the natural flow of nature to help us in all our endeavors.

IN THE ZONE

Athletes have always known the elevated feeling when they are "in the zone." It is the feeling of being in effortless flow, as if the action were doing itself. A ball player knows it when he or she hits the ball just right and they "feel" the home run before the ball leaves the bat. Teachers and public speakers feel the zone when it seems as if the words just come out perfectly on their own. Dancers are in the zone when they perform and feel as if they were watching themselves go through the routines.

> **Procedure**. In the next several weeks, be observant of your feelings while performing your duties, sport, or job. Try to notice when you fall into an effortless flow of doing. In most cases it will be with something you are very familiar with or something you are extremely good at doing. Also notice the effect of any effort or trying while performing your activity. In fact, just your added effort or judgmental attention will change the flow feeling. When you can start to have this

feeling and effortlessness in most of your activity, you will come to understand what the Tai Chi and Qigong Masters experience daily.

THE THREE MOST IMPORTANT WORDS....

When I first met Shifu Jiang Jian-ye, who was to become my Tai Chi Master for many years, I moved respectfully to the back of the class and awaited instruction. His good-natured charm was a delight to see, but this was matched by his quiet display of tremendous internal strength, which seemed to emanate from his mid-section. I was impressed before the first words left his mouth. But what he had to say to us was equally impressive, and it remains a corner stone of the teaching and practice. And what did he say?

The three most important words in Tai Chi (and Qigong): first word—relax. The second word—relax. Third word—relax.

I was to later learn that relaxation comes in layers. Deeper relaxation necessitated more intricate or subtle techniques. Much of Western calisthenics involves tightening and a forced effort. Here we were asked to move, but move with relaxation, so as to allow the energy lines or meridians to stay dilated, and thus provide for greater internal energy flow. Once I truly understood this concept, the principles and particulars of Tai Chi and Qigong practice became clear.

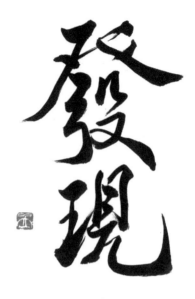

3

HOW TO APPROACH A TREE

"Can't see the forest for the trees?" Trees, like humans, rarely live alone. Trees of like species are, in fact, families. They live in communities, connected by their roots, and actually communicate, according to Peter Wohlleben in *The Hidden Life of Trees. (3)*

In the forest the crisscross of tree energies or auras forms a web-like invisible mesh. As we slowly make our way down the wooded path, we unknowingly pass through this vast energetic field. It bathes us, soothes the system, and brings a healing shawl of energy all around us. The ancient Taoists advised us to "breathe the air of trees"—air that is rich in anti-oxidants, oxygen, and negative ions. Were it a pill, it would be worth everything.

Look to the trees, children. In their stillness, they give to us. Cut off a limb, and they still give us fruit. Be like that tree—silent, service, beauty.

Amma Karunamayi

As you approach the forest or park, become silent. In your stillness, begin to sense your surroundings. Establish that you are here now in this moment and begin to feel, see, and hear. Does one tree attract you more than others? Or do you feel drawn to a portion of the forest or park, not yet explored? Step into the present moment and get in touch with your inner body—feel the skin, feel the whole body. Allow the body to become like a powerful receptor. Allow the energies of the whole forest or a particular tree to actually pull you.

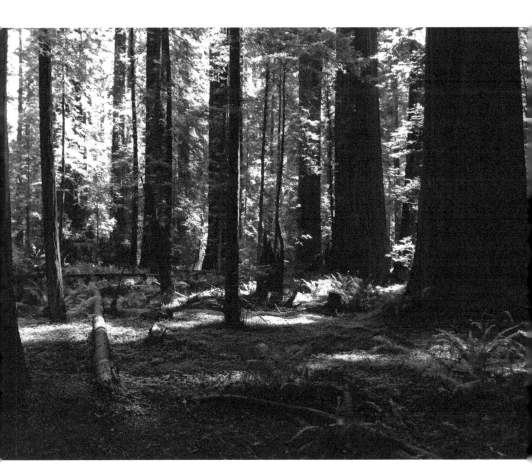

ENTER THE FOREST

This "approach experience" could be in the form of seeing a tree that is simply beautiful or one of feeling the tree energetically pulling you closer. The key to finding a good tree to work with is being present and feeling your body. With such stillness and awareness we become aware of something sacred, as if the tree you choose has wonderful, deep secrets to explore. Let the tree reciprocate. Imagine your tree is feeling your sacredness, your latent Divinity. Put aside your worries and problems. Leave them at the forest edge. Energize your receptors and remain open .

A simple procedure as you approach the forest

1. Establish present moment awareness by feeling your own body, feel your own inner energy field.
2. Check to see if you are holding tension or tightness. Scan your body and let go, profoundly relax.
3. As you maintain this subtle body feeling, bring your attention to the forest, park, or particular tree.
4. Become still and engage an inner smile.
5. Then simply let the right tree pull you. Let your intuition or feeling level take over.

The simple act of putting your attention on your body or inner energy field anchors you to the present moment. It is in this space that tree or forest energy can be perceived—certainly not in thoughts about future or past events.

Tightness in the body is often the result of stress, congestion, or constriction. Let the body settle and feel the weight of gravity without fighting it. Feel as if your bones were mere coat hangers and your muscles were coats, draped easily over them. This will facilitate the feeling of letting go, producing more relaxation.

With this relaxed present moment body awareness, simply add

the additional awareness of your forest surroundings. Be aware of your body and, at the same time, be aware of the nature in front of you. Approach the tree as you would start a Tai Chi Form or classical recital.

The Inner Smile

The inner smile is a tool used for inner relaxation and healing. The Taoist Masters say that the inner smile can be the doorway to the inner realms. When we are aware of the forest with an inner smile, nature smiles back. We feel a comfort, a kinship. Here is the beginning of what the Masters call connectedness—a realization that the energy within us is intimately connected to the energy outside of us. It leads to the experience of enlightenment, a cosmic unity.

We use the inner smile to open that door. Smile to nature and she will lead you—this is the approach.

Another method is to engage the heart. Simple move your awareness to the heart place and feel as if the heart is actually breathing in the air around you. This will anchor you to the heart, that place the Taoist Masters would often call the "Emperor of the Emotions." From this heart center use your feelings to find the tree that will work best for you. In this tender feeling place, it may very well be that the tree will find you!

Being led to a particular kind of tree, or one that just feels right is the first stage. As you get closer, be even more sensitive to your own body sensations. Does the tree feel hot, cool, prickly, or pleasant? Simply be aware of the "too's." Check inside and see if the tree energy is too hot, too cold, too strong, too powerful. You are seeking a tree that feels pleasant to you.

Begin to think of your chosen tree as a "thou," and not an "it." Give your tree sentience, feeling, and wisdom—even a personality.

BIG TREE, LITTLE TREE

Energy from trees practice is ancient. The Taoists have been practicing this way for centuries. There are records of tree practices that go back to the Yellow Emperor 2700 B.C. As these techniques and philosophy pass down through the ages, they are interpreted and taught by the Masters.

My first fascination with tree energy came after I began to work with multiple masters over a number of years: Shifu Jiang Jian-Ye, Mantak Chia, Master Lee Holden, and Dr. Yang Jwing Ming. I became particularly interested in "energy from trees" practices, due to a lifelong love of nature, forests, and wooded countryside. I began to discover that each Master had a different approach, a different way to getting this energy. They did not contradict each other, but complimented each other. Their varied approaches were simply different layers or ways to absorb that same energy. Instead of having to decide which approach to take, it became both fascinating and rewarding to use these different techniques in concert. My "toolbox" of tree energy methods became full, and I had multiple approaches from which to pull. In fact, I was to soon discover, each different tree or trip to the forest allowed me a chance to choose the approach. Was I going to find a five-element tree today for my liver function or perhaps I simply needed to recharge the system? Did I need to let the tree and sun take my excess stagnant energy, or did I simply need Mother Nature's comfort that day? At times it is good to allow the trees to make that choice. At times it is good to allow the trees to make that choice. Some Masters encourage the use of large trees to absorb abundant energy. Others prefer smaller, younger trees because they're hungry for your energy and would gladly give you theirs.

There is a hidden subtle energy life in the forest, in trees. To enter this energy field is to enter a world of profound depth, expanse, and beauty. It is often perceived as something with a vast field of mystery and enchantment, and yet something that is intimately connected to your own being.

In Short...

Approaching a tree is much like finding a friend. You simply need to have intention. Perhaps the right tree will find you! Trees use our energy as we use theirs. It is a mutual friendship—we have much to learn from each other.

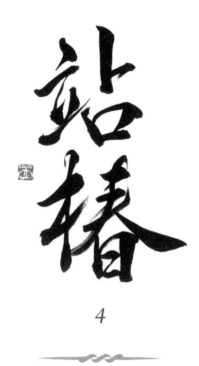

4

ABSORBING TREE ENERGY

The practice of absorbing energy from trees is at the heart of the Five Element Orchard system of Qigong. There are estimated to be over three thousand different styles of Qigong being practiced today. It is a very common occurrence to see people practicing one or more of these styles throughout Asia in city parks in the morning. Qigong is gaining popularity in the United States, as practitioners in increasing numbers are finding the benefits of these ancient practices. These different styles have a wide range of movement and method, ranging from strong energy workouts to simply standing still. Workouts can include single movements arranged for purposes of gaining and circulating energy, as well as specific sets of moves such as the popular "Eight Pieces of Brocade." Qigong is sometimes also taught in dance-like patterns that allow for a greater flow of energy in the body. These graceful forms often follow the movements of animals, real or mythological.

However, all Qigong movement targets the use of energy—energy that can be stored, generated and circulated throughout the body—or taken, or borrowed, from the atmosphere around us.

To successfully absorb energy from trees, we need to borrow techniques from a number of Qigong styles. One of the most powerful systems of energy practice is one with the least amount of movement. Standing poses, a Qigong called Zhan Zhuang, is an ancient practice that has its roots in stillness. Pronounced "Jam Jong," the name Zhan Zhuang, interestingly enough, is often translated as "Standing Like a Tree." We also need to go to those Qigong practices that emphasize the importance of breathing. In Traditional Chinese Medicine there is an emphasis on how energy travels or circulates throughout the system. This includes an understanding that there are special places on the body where there is more electromagnetic energy called acupressure or acupuncture points. A few of these special areas on the body serve as "gates" where energy can easily travel in and out of the system.

STANDING POSES FOR ABSORBING
THE ENERGY OF TREES

Qigong stances develop strength. Holding a stance in an aligned manner allows you to put very mild tension into a part of the body while relaxing and breathing deeply at the same time. This allows you to open the meridian channels, encouraging energy to move through the system easily. This circulation of energy, or Qi, helps to remove stagnant blockages and provide healing for areas in need.

A stance with proper body alignment also allows you to connect with earth energy. A prolonged holding of the stance gives you the opportunity to feel rooted into the earth and, at the same time, feel a cooling, transforming energy come into the body. Earth energy is considered cool, magnetic, and grounding.

The stationary experience of holding the stance gives you the opportunity to "listen" to your inner body. You have the opportunity to strengthen and develop a greater sensitivity to the internal energies that travel through the system. This experience quickly develops the ability to sense energy blockages and energy deficiencies. With this inner knowing you can direct the energy to flow appropriately.

In another way, the practice of holding stances in Qigong gives you the opportunity to stop, if only for a moment, the incessant momentum of movement and activity that propels us throughout the day. We begin to instill the mind with a sense of emptiness. We step into the present moment, withholding both thought and movement. With this habit, we begin to move towards an awareness that helps us to develop a strong spiritual foundation.

THE IDEAL METAPHOR

As previously mentioned, the tree becomes the ideal metaphor for how energy works in the body. The tree also becomes an excellent metaphor for how to stand. As we align our body, we align our meridians to insure the smooth flow of energy throughout the system. We virtually become a conduit for bio-electromagnetic energy running through the body. If properly aligned, we feel the flood of energy throughout the body as if it has suddenly become alive, buzzing with Qi.

Three ingredients are necessary for these stances to produce their magic:

1. **Relaxation**. This is most easily accomplished by proper breathing. Long, slow, continuous breathing will calm the body down and relax muscular tension and any tightness due to stress factors. The body must be free of all tension or tightness in order to feel relaxed, comfortable, and balanced.

2. **Attention**. Our attention needs to be on the body. The energy will go where our mind goes. In many stances, the simple

act of placing our attention on the lower Tan Tien or abdomen has many benefits. If we are working on a particular organ, or five-element association to that organ, our attention needs to be there.

3. **Proper alignment**. Our bodies must be properly aligned (see "The Three Powers Position"). We must create the conditions for a free flow of energy from earth and the heavens by aligning and straightening the meridian lines.

THE THREE POWERS POSE

The first preparatory stance is often called "The Three Powers Pose" in China. This is because it is an excellent metaphor for the three primordial powers of heaven, human, and earth. Heaven energy could be described as "electric," as it is projecting, powerful and moving—this is Yang energy. Whereas, earth energies are measured as magnetic or condensing and sinking—this is Yin energy. Human energy is innate, generated within the body in three major energy centers called Tan Tiens or Elixir Fields.

Thus, the "Three Powers Position" is a stance that contains or houses what the scientific community would call bio-electromagnetic energy.

This simple standing position aligns the meridians, allowing energy to ascend into the system from earth and come desend into the system from the heavens, gathering in the lower tan tien in the area of the abdomen.

The Three Powers Stance takes its name and inspiration from the tree itself. Trees also seek these same energies. The canopies reach upward and, at the same time, trees sink their roots deep into the earth. Tree energy runs through the cambia underneath the bark and out to each limb and leaf.

Practicing "The Three Powers Pose"

- Stand with your feet shoulder width apart with both feet flat to the floor or ground, weight evenly distributed.
- Make the knees "soft," not bent or locked at attention.
- Allow your attention to come up to the waist and tuck the sacrum down and in slightly.
- Slightly spread the scapula in the upper back and allow your shoulders to round forward slightly. This will produce a space in the armpits, as your arms hang down at the sides like loose ropes.
- Pull the chin in and allow the neck to lengthen. This should allow the very top of the head to point straight upwards.
- All these micro movements will allow energy coming from earth and heaven to move through the meridian lines with significantly reduced obstruction.
- Allow your arms to gently lift into an embracing position at chest level. Feel as if you are actually holding something to your chest.
- Now relax into this pose and let go of any tensions or restrictions you may feel.

With this practice you are mirroring the "movement" of the tree. You allow your crown point to feel as if connected to the sun and all the heaven energies. At the same time, you mentally sink into the earth, producing a sense of rooting. This practice will help you to feel centered and balanced.

The Three Powers Pose becomes the starting template for a number of specific stances, which will help us to direct tree energy to different parts of the body and organs.

Please note: *These particular stances are for absorbing energy from trees. In chapter six you will also find additional stances to absorb the energy of specific tree odors.*

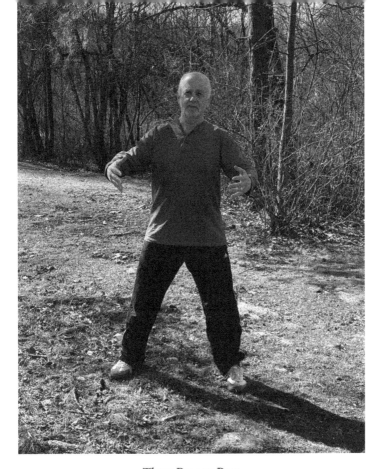

Three Powers Pose

GRATITUDE AND THE INNER SMILE

In all the following tree poses or stances, you will be asked to get in touch with the energy of your chosen tree. This means you must still your mind and put your attention on the tree in a loving way. Two things that can help this process are the feeling of gratitude and the practice of engaging a subtle inner smile. As you work with your tree, be grateful for all its life-giving properties, as well as its beauty and charm. See each tree as having a personality and a heartbeat. Be grateful that these swaying giants are on this planet to help and heal you. They are here for you. They love you. Return the favor. Also use a subtle warm inner smile coming from your heart. As previously mentioned, this will help you to relax and sense the tree's energy more clearly, as well as provide a way for the tree to feel your loving energy.

The main practice with these stances is simply to stand and relax. Additional activities include some gentle movements, which will allow you to feel the tree's energy. In each pose you will also be asked to breathe deeply, allowing the tree's individual odor to absorb into the body. This is a significant part of the practice, as the ancient Masters held that the odor of the tree was the most potent elixir of all.

FEELING TREE ENERGY WITH MOVEMENT

This is a general tree pose with movements for feeling tree energy. It can be used with any tree for any physical or emotional concern. In this particular stance we will be adding gentle movements designed to gather and feel the tree's energy field.

The Basic Stance

Stand facing the tree, feet together. Then open your feet to shoulder-width. Bring your arms up with the trunk between the hands, palms facing the tree. As with all of the Five Element Orchard practices, you do not touch the tree, but hold your palms one to four inches away in order to feel the tree's energy with greater sensitivity and subtlety.

Additional Movements

Sliding Up and Down. Keeping the arms and palms in a steady position, slowly lower and raise the body by bending at the knees. Do not touch the tree, but feel the tree energy and your hands move up and down along the bark as you go down and up. Repeat 36 times.

Forward and Back. Next, lean the upper body forward and then back so the palms move back and forth, with the trunk between them. Do not shift the hips forward and backward. Note that this

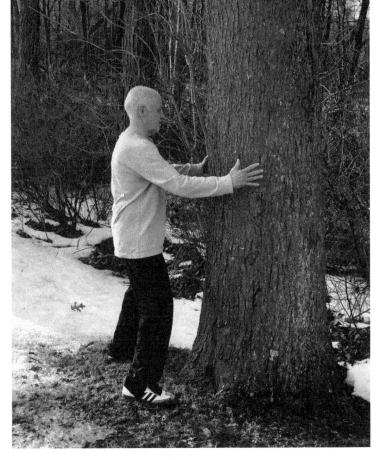

Feeling Tree Energy

pose is similar to the Three Powers Pose, but now with subtle added movements. Repeat 36 times.

Rotation. With this movement you will gently rotate your palms around the tree as if loosening a huge jar. You can move both ways. Repeat 36 times

TREE POSE FOR THE LUNGS

In Chinese Five Element Theory the lungs are associated with the heavy emotions, such as anxiety, depression, grief, and loss. The lungs are said to be the "commanders of Qi." This pose allows you to sense and feel tree energy and then direct it to the lungs and surrounding areas. This increased energy not only works on the lungs on an emotional level, but also on a physical level, bringing more life-giving tree energy to the lungs and related disorders.

1. Stand close to your chosen tree, a little less than arms-length away. Align the body as outlined in "The Three Powers Pose." Hold your arms straight out as if to embrace the tree, so that both palms face the sides of the trunk (a few inches away). The tree trunk is then between your palms. Now, lower your palms along the trunk to waist level. You will note that this pose is similar to the previous standing position, but

Lung Pose

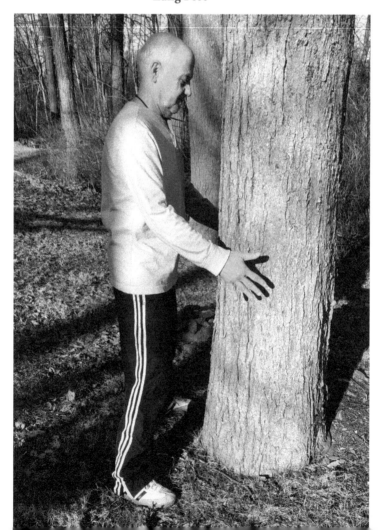

the difference here is where we hold our attention—in this case, the lungs and surrounding area. Remember, energy goes where your attention goes. First, feel the tree energy and then direct it to the lungs.

2. Thank the tree for allowing you to embrace it and receive. Breath deeply, as you get in touch with the feeling of the tree's energy, odor, and healing properties.

3. Rotate or Twist Qi. Use the whole body to rotate energy around the tree, first one way and then the other. This will look as if you are trying to twist a jar lid loose with both hands. Do this one way and then the other. Do not touch the tree. Repeat 36 times.

4. Now breathe deeply as you take in the odor of the tree, and allow the lungs to absorb this health giving-elixir.

5. Thank your lungs for breathing "twenty-four seven" for you. Again, thank the tree and slowly come back to a normal stance.

Tree Pose for the Kidneys

When the lungs take in Qi from the air that we breath, Traditional Chinese Medicine tells us that the kidneys grab this energy and move it throughout the body. The kidneys are connected to our ability to feel at ease and free from fear. Bringing energy to this part of the body also helps numerous digestive and elimination disorders.

1. Approach your tree with gratitude and reverence. Align your body as in "The Three Powers Pose."

2. Turn around, so that the trunk of the tree is behind you.

3. Bend the knees and bend forward slightly, as you move your arms behind you. Place both palms on either side of the trunk behind you. Make sure you have the tree trunk between your two palms or as close as you can.

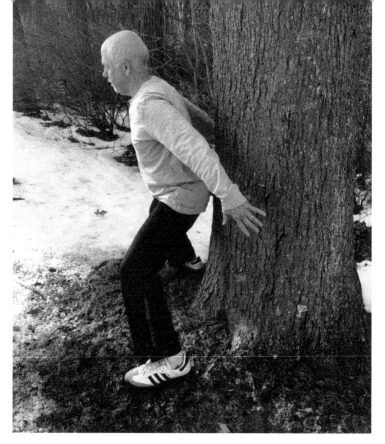

Kidney Pose

4. Bring Qi from the tree to the Ming-Men (kidney area). Circle the arms around behind the body, reaching toward the tree, then bring them back toward the body with palms facing the kidney area. Exhale as you reach toward the tree and inhale as hands come back toward the body. Repeat 3 times.

5. Now place your attention on the kidneys as you breathe. Feel the tree's power infuse your kidneys with life-giving, healing energy. See if you can distinguish the tree's particular life-giving odor.

6. Thank the tree for allowing you to embrace it and receive its energy. Breathe deeply as you get in touch with the feeling of tree's energy, odor, and healing properties.

TREE POSE FOR THE LIVER

The liver, our largest internal organ, has a close relationship with the blood. As much as a fourth of our blood supply can be in the liver at any given time. In Traditional Chinese Medicine the liver is said to house anger, resentment, and jealousy. When nourished and bathed in Qi the energetic emotional transformation is to a positive feeling of kindness.

1. Approach your tree with gratitude and reverence. Align your body as in "The Three Powers Pose."
2. Next stand in a "Forward stance" with the right leg forward and slightly bent. The rear left leg is straighter. Cradle the trunk of the tree between your palms.
3. As you feel the energy of the tree between your hands,

Liver Pose

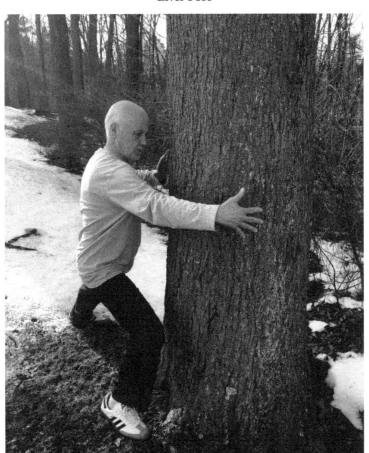

imagine you are pushing Qi from your left hand to the right hand through the tree. As the energy goes into your right palm, feel it travel up that arm and down to the liver on your right side of your floating rib area. Allow the liver to fill up with the power of life-giving tree energy.

4. Thank the tree for allowing you to embrace it and receive its energy. Breathe deeply into the liver, as you get in touch with the feeling of the tree's energy, odor, and healing properties.

5. Thank your liver for all it does to process your blood, food and energy for you. Again thank the tree and slowly come back to a normal stance.

Tree Pose for the Heart

In Traditional Chinese Medicine the heart is considered the emperor of the emotions. Western scientists are now discovering that the heart area has the strongest electromagnetic force in the body. We literally project who we really are to the world through the heart. This organ is a great receiver and sender of energy. The heart can hold hatred and resentment as well as love and forgiveness. Fresh vibrant energy can be the agent of change from the negative emotion to the positive.

1. Approach your tree with gratitude and reverence. Align your body as in "The Three Powers Pose."

2. Thank the tree for allowing you to embrace it and receive. Breathe deeply as you get in touch with the feeling of the tree's energy, odor, and healing properties.

3. Slowly raise both your palms upward, facing the tree's trunk. Reach up so that your palms extend up the tree above the level of your head.

4. Feel the energy of the tree and channel this force down your arms to the area of the heart. Keep your hands facing the tree trunk, but put your attention on the heart. Energy goes where your attention goes.

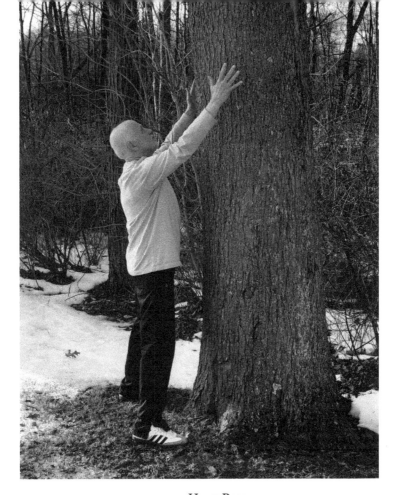

Heart Pose

5. Thank the tree for allowing you to embrace it and receive its energy. Breathe deeply into the heart.
6. Thank your heart for beating twenty-four seven, providing you with life. Thank the tree again and slowly come back to a normal standing pose.

TREE POSE FOR THE SPLEEN

Taoist masters have always known that the spleen is closely related to the stomach; consequently, it plays an important part in digestion. In this tradition it is the spleen that extracts the energy from the food we eat and disseminates it throughout the body. The spleen harbors our worry and rumination, and positive energy transmutes these emotions to balance and provide a feeling of centeredness.

1. This pose is basically the same as the tree pose for the liver, but on the other side.
2. In this pose feel the energy of the tree and push this energy with the right hand into the left palm into the spleen on the left side of your abdomen.
3. Breathe the fragrance of your tree and thank your tree and spleen for what they do for you.
4. Thank your tree for giving its life-supporting energy to important parts of your body and healing mental and physical concerns.

Spleen Pose

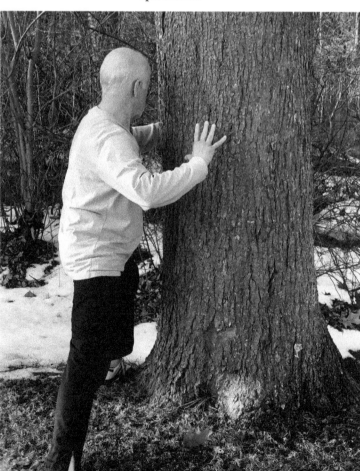

TREE ENERGY FOR THE SENSES

Stand facing the tree with arms extended so that each palm is facing the two sides of the tree. Bring Qi from the tree. Without touching the tree, the hands frame around the trunk and inhale. Then move hands from the tree, palms down, to just above the bai hui (the crown point at the top of the head) as you exhale. Now hold this position and inhale and exhale. Repeat three times. Similar exercises can be done by bringing Qi from the tree to the eyes, nose, mouth and ears, while inhaling and exhaling.

Bring Tree Energy to the Senses

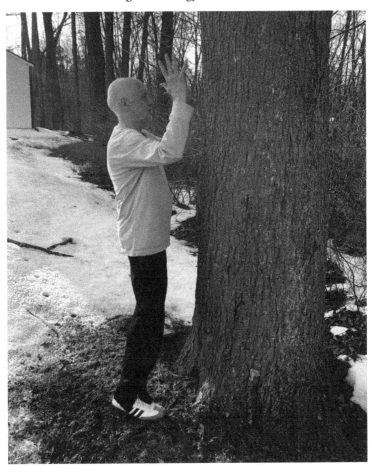

Tree Energy for the Tan Tien
(The Body's Energy Center)

Stand facing the tree with arms extended. Bring tree Qi to the Tan Tien (abdominal area). Hold palms in front of the lower abdomen, palms facing in. Circle arms out and away from body toward tree, then in a scooping motion bring palms back to the lower abdomen. Exhale as hands move toward the tree and inhale as they move toward the body. Repeat three more times.

What Does Tree Energy Feel Like?

Each individual will experience tree energy differently. This is a world of subtle vibration. How one perceives its sensations and movement will vary from individual to individual, but other variants include time of day, outside temperature, etc.

In addition, and perhaps most importantly, tree energy will feel differently with different trees. Don't expect the giant oak to feel like a smaller willow. In general, however, most people tend to feel tree energy as one or more of these sensations: warm, soft, spongy, thick, buzzing, tingly. At times it may be a slight vibration and at other times is can be incredibly powerful. Look for changes in temperature, sensation, and feeling. You may have to be with the tree for a while before you experience a discernable feeling. Relax, let go of tensions in the body, and breathe.

Alternative Methods for
Gathering Tree Energy

The following techniques and procedures are additional methods of absorbing energy from trees. They can be used individually or in concert with each other. With experience and experimentation, you can find the ones that work best for you. In all procedures we can use the following sequence:

1. Find the tree with which you wish to work. You can be guided by your intuition or look for the right tree according to the Five Element Orchard design described in Chapter Six. Remember that Oak trees and Pines trees are giants of energy, prolific, and are always a good choice if you are unsure.

2. Approach your tree with reverence and gratitude. Ask your tree permission to absorb its energy, as you would ask a wise old man or saintly woman. Understand that you are about to engage in a wonderful exchange—an exchange on a very subtle, yet powerful level. Trees have always known the importance of deep rooting and connecting to the heavens. Their patience is endless and their language is one of silence. Approach humbly, with a willingness to learn from them.

3. Engage in the appropriate stance around the tree, be silent, breathe deeply and try to let go of tensions and worries of the day. You have come here for peace—welcome it.

4. Use one or more methods of taking in tree energy. Experiment.

5. Once you feel the tree energy, especially in your palms, place and keep your attention on the organ or part of the body where you want this energy to go. Let the tree's subtle vibrations enter this area.

6. Stay with this experience for a while, knowing that it is healing on many levels. You will leave the forest or park with energy from the trees—vibrant, fresh, clean.

7. When you feel it is time, move away from your tree, simultanously thanking your tree for the exchange.

USING ENERGY GATES FOR ABSORBING TREE ENERGY

Trees and the human body are two of nature's powerhouses of energy, both having the ability to give and receive Qi, internal energy.

In essence we could say that we are enacting a reciprocal agreement to exchange energy with trees. They use our CO_2, what we perceive as old or stagnant energy, and we feel the benefit of oxygen rich energy from them. How can we best absorb what trees have to give us? The answer is literally in our hands!

Previously, we learned that the body is a conduit between heaven and earth forces. When channeled, these forces surge through our systems, providing energy and health. Our bodies have "gates," special points on the body, that can be used to bring this energy into the system. Earth energy is cooling, grounding, and centering. It is the earth that can also absorb our negative, stale or old energy. Energies from the heavens are more electric, powerful, and expanding. We are going to add tree energy to these earth and cosmic power sources

To accommodate this constant flow of energy from earth and the cosmos, the human nervous system is equipped with energy points or vortexes that act like doorways, letting energy in and energy out. Although energy enters and leaves our bodies through our breath, skin, and even our pores, there are three special "gates" that can process large amounts of energies.

The acupressure point on the bottom of the foot, (the first point on the kidney meridian) Kidney 1 (K1), is an area where we take energy in from earth. A proper stance, attention and relaxation are the keys for this energy infusion to happen.

Conversely, the crown point (GV 20) at the top of the head acts like a gate to the cosmos, allowing energy in from the planets, sun, moon, and the galaxies. When Tai Chi practitioners perform their slow, relaxed movements, they are often taught to feel the "heavenly pull," or feeling, that a silent force is gently tugging them up, producing greater alignment and a feeling of being connected to heaven forces.

However, the two points on the hands near the center of the palms are truly unique "gates," due to their versatility. These points are on the pericardium meridian (P8) and are called Laogong, or "Palace of Weariness." Their versatility lies in the mobility of the hands—we can point these gates to earth, to the heavens, to our body or another person for healing. We can use these gates to absorb tree energy.

The power comes when we place these points towards each other. In doing so, we create a current of energy similar to an electric charge. Your hands become conduits of energy or like two terminals or poles of an electric current. With practice, relaxed attention, and an increased awareness of our connections to earth and heaven forces, this charge becomes stronger, and the number of uses for the energy is endless. Qigong masters use these two palm points for healing, simply by placing one palm on one side of the part of the body, that is injured (the knee, for example), and the other palm on the other side. The cross current enters the body, allowing life force energy to flow into the area in need.

We can also extract both positive and negative energies with these two points. When absorbing energy from trees, we simply place one palm on one side of the trunk of the tree and the other palm on the opposite side of the truck. Instantly, a subtle cross current is created. With each tree practice session, this current gets noticeably stronger. When these palm points are used with specific breathing techniques and proper stances, tree energy can be absorbed and directed to a particular area, or to one of the five "life" organs (lungs, kidneys, liver, heart, and spleen).

Wave Hands

Simply hold the hands on either side of the trunk and gently wave them towards you, as if you were wafting the aroma of your favorite soup to your nose. We "waft" the tree energy to the desired organ or body part. Along with the use of one of several standing poses, energy is gently directed to a specific organ.

BREATHING FOR ENERGY ABSORPTION

As long ago as two thousand years, early Taoist healers knew about one of the most powerful medicines in all of nature—the aroma coming from trees. Medical prescriptions often included the addition of "breathe the air of trees." It is the odor or aroma of trees that penetrates into your system, not only nourishing the brain through the nose, but affecting all parts of the body. And these Masters knew through experimentation, deep meditation, and contemplation, how certain tree odors affect different life organs, and consequently, different emotions. To walk through a heavily wooded area, is to walk through nature's pharmacy!

To fully absorb this life-giving elixir, however, appropriate breathing methods are needed.

Abdominal Breathing

Gently place both your hands over your stomach area, just below the belly button.

Slowly inhale deep into the lungs, so as to have the feeling that you are filling up a balloon in your abdomen. Breathe through the nose and only take in about 80% of your lung capacity. When you exhale through the nose, have the feeling that your imaginary balloon is slowly deflating. Your breath should be long, slow, deep, and continuous. Continue to inhale and exhale through the nose in this fashion for a few minutes.

Your almost immediate experience will be one of settling down and relaxation. By breathing into the lower lobes of the lungs, you are starting to activate the parasympathetic nervous system, that part of your autonomic system that tells the body that you are safe, not in danger, and you can heal. When you breathe the air of trees, this calming feeling is enhanced.

Three-Part Breathing or "Wave Breath"

This breathing method is really a continuation of normal abdominal breathing. We breathe into the belly as before, but now continue the in-breath to fill up the chest area and then the upper clavicle area. This is done with a smooth, continuous in-breath. With this wave like intake of air the spine begins to bend and flow gently like soft whip. Breathing into the abdominal area brings relaxation, while the breath into the upper lung area creates an alertness in the mind. The whole process gently creates a "restful alertness." As with abdominal breathing, your breathing should be long, slow, deep and continuous.

Skin Breathing

This is a wonderful breathing exercise that can be done anytime in Nature. Although it relies on a degree of imagination, the experience is strong and often described as, "it seems as if my whole body is breathing." Find an enjoyable place to stand that feels good to you: on a forest path, in a grove of trees, in a meadow, and so forth. Stand in the Wuji stance previously mentioned and breathe normally for a few breaths. Then bring your attention to the whole body and imagine that when you breathe in, the air is coming in through every cell of you body, as if every cell on your skin were taking in the oxygen. When you exhale, feel as if any toxicity is leaving your body through the pores. This is a truly liberating experience in a wooded area. We literally "feel" the forest coming in, hugging the body.

The "No-Breath Breathing" Technique

No-breath breathing is a unique form of absorbing both oxygen and Qi into the body. You initiate this procedure by breathing in through the nose slowly. With both your intention and attention, pull in tree energy as the breath comes in. Breathe in only half of your breath, stopping the incoming air but continue with a mental drawing in of the energy, as if you were sucking in more energy with a gentle tightening of the lungs. The first half of the breath draws in oxygen. When you stop the in-breath, the Qi continues to come in and your mind is more silent and freer to actually observe this intake of energy. You literally suck it into the system. It is recommended that you do this for no longer than three to six breaths, as longer periods may feel like you are straining the musculature around the lungs. It is in the second half of this breath that we take in the energy deeply. If the no-breath breathing method feels awkward or a strain, simply leave out the second part and absorb the tree energy with the full in-breath through the nose. We will add a unique hand motion called "Octopus Fingers" to this breathing method.

OCTOPUS FINGERS

This hand movement technique, that is used in conjunction with breathing methods, uses the Pericardium 8 point in the center of the palm. We want to draw in tree energy into these points of both hands. To do this we simply pull the palms slowly away from the tree, as we gently close the fingers—as if the fingers were tongs pulling spaghetti out of the pan. In fact, that "something" is energy that we pull out of the tree with the hands. We pull the energy from the tree as the fingers gently close together—like an octopus!

Combining No-breath Breathing with
Octopus Fingers and Stance

Combining the breath work and hand movements, while standing near a chosen tree, you are able to access the power, the energy of the tree. This tree energy can then be directed to particular parts of the body or organ for healing and health maintenance. In a subsequent chapter we will discuss which trees have energy that can work well with specific organs in the body for health and healing purposes. Apply the no-breath breathing method as you move the hands away from the tree and, at the same time, use the "octopus" hand movements. The combination of no-breath breathing and octopus fingers has a magical effect.

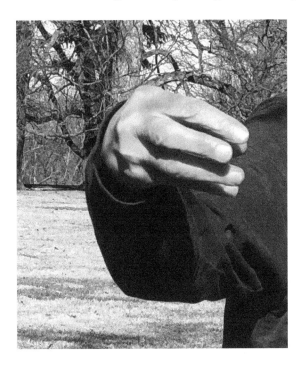

BREATHING THE AIR OF TREES

Many of the breathing methods mentioned can be done in conjunction with the stances or can be practiced on their own. One effective method of using breathing methods for absorbing energy from trees is to find a large tree that you feel comfortable with and make sure that you stand under the canopy of the tree, so that you have the tree surrounding you, so to speak. This is a great way to absorb energy by taking in tree aroma and energy. We are truly breathing the air of trees!

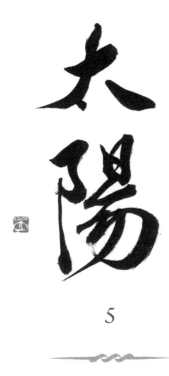

5

FOLLOW THE SUN

The day of the sun is like the day of a king. It is a promenade in the morning, a sitting on the throne at noon, a pageant in the evening. (1)

Wallace Stevens

So powerful, so life giving, and so important to life on the planet is the Sun. In Hinduism the Sun is considered God. Also known as Surya, this God is the creator of the universe and the source of all life. Surya is considered the supreme soul who brings light and warmth to the world. Surya is worshipped across the Indian subcontinent and is also a minor deity in Buddhism.

In the Vedic ritual, Surya Namaskara, practitioners awaken early

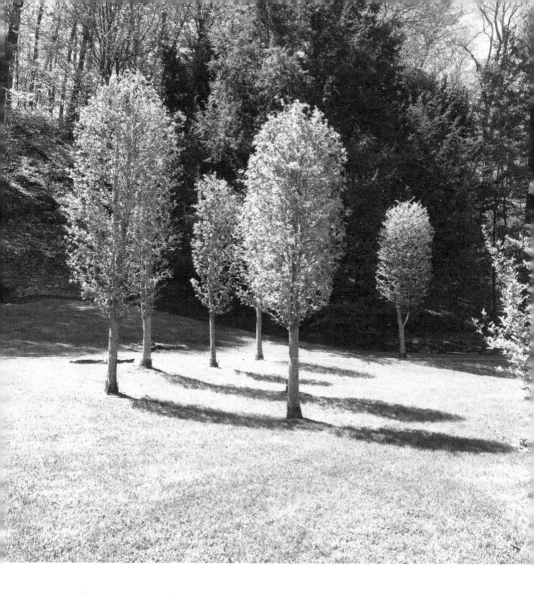

and go outside to face the eastern rising sun to absorb the solar energy emanating from the golden rays. The early rising Sun is considered especially powerful and life-giving. This time is considered a cosmic time for Qi, as it floods into the body, charging up the subtle energy centers in the system. Vedic practitioners see the Sun God as a wonderful boon for health, a natural treasure that can awaken dormant energy and heal all wounds.

The Taoists have long believed that we all possess a body of light,

THE FIVE ELEMENT ORCHARD

that we are light at our very core. The light that illuminates the universe is our light. Your body of light is where your consciousness resonates with the energy of the universe. This light within helps all levels of life. Physical healing, inner balance and a sense of excitement, mental clarity, open mindedness, and a feeling of expansion are all a result of the light we possess within. When our body is perfectly balanced and refined, our internal energy will start to become illuminated, and our body of light shines forth. In spiritual Qigong the practitioner seeks to connect to a higher force. We seek to experience our body of light that can connect us to the Tao, our higher self.

We need to raise the frequency of our energy to match the energy of nature. When energy is distilled to a higher frequency, we start to experience an inner alchemy. Stress turns to vitality, negative emotions turn to positive, and the wandering mind turns to wisdom.

Cultivating our body of light brings in an awareness or feeling of a connection to a higher power and the entire universe.

From where comes such a rich source of energy and light? The greatest source of energy outside the body is the sun, or electromagnetic radiation. Light is energy, and we need to cultivate it. All of life benefits from the Sun. Even the food we eat for sustenance comes from the Sun. Plants are stored sunlight—they transfer sunlight through photosynthesis. We get sunlight through plants we eat. Even animals eat the plants and transfer that energy to us when we ingest this kind of protein. We constantly take light into the body through the air that we breathe, the food that we eat, and the water we drink. Our bodies are "light driven."

If we acknowledge plant life to be a rich source of light and, therefore, life itself, what then of trees? If the salad we eat at lunch gives life-giving light, what power, what magnificent source of energy must exist in those giants that rise ever towards the source of light, the sun. When we consider the rich solar energy within that beautiful maple tree, tapping the tree for its sap seems a far lesser yield than the rich sun energy it also has for us.

Face the South Side of the Tree

Getting energy from trees is absorbing its electromagnetic radiation, its stored sunlight. To do this we simply need to observe the tree's ever thirst for sunlight—the canopy ever reaching towards the sun, as it opens its leaves to receive this source. During the day, the tree's energy, its focus so to speak, is ever upwards towards the source of light. However, we know that the sun travels a southerly route (in the northern hemisphere), and if you look at a cross section of the tree trunk, you will notice a series of rings that tend to move more to one side. And we learned as school children that the rings, in most species, identify the age of the tree. What we may not have been taught or realized is that the rings are never perfectly circular, that they "bulge" to one side. It will come as no surprise at this point that the rings tend to move towards the south side facing the sun, indicating how trees are ever leaning and absorbing this form of electromagnetic energy. It should also come as no surprise that the south side of the tree contains the most solar energy, the most power.

However, standing on the west side of the tree at sunset has its value if the practitioner wants to reduce excess energy. If one is too excited or too emotional, the west side of a tree at sunset will pull that energy down with the sun.

Use the Dusk and Dawn Hours

When the sun begins to set, the energy of the tree starts to move downward towards the roots. In the night hours the strongest energy comes from below. The root system absorbs, uses, and sends the energy of nutrients from earth. Trees give off their strongest healing odor at dusk. You may even feel a little dizzy at this time if you are in a deeply wooded area or perhaps a slight oppression due to over-oxygenation. At dusk the sunlight has left and the botanically nutrient rich tree odors come down to the lower part of the tree due to

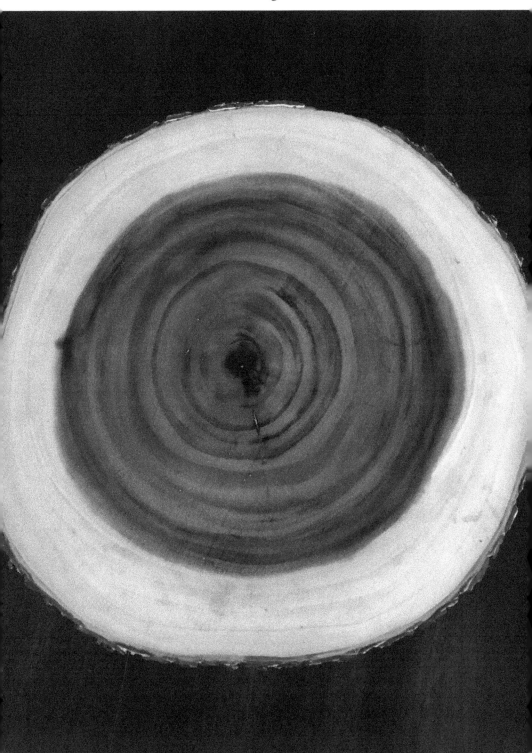

the gravitational pull to earth. The atmosphere becomes more dense, with relatively little carbon dioxide, but rich in oxygen. When we practice in a forest environment, we absorb these nutrients that destroy bacteria, viruses, and other pathogens. Trees become our pharmacy. Just breathe!

There is this shifting of energy from canopy to roots and roots to canopy, a continuous flow of Qi from the sun and Qi from earth.

We cannot stand in the canopy in midday, nor can we go to the roots in the evening. But we can stand at the trunk. Standing at the trunk becomes particularly significant and valuable when we realize that the energy is at trunk level in the transition times. In other words, energy descends down from the canopy as the sun sets and rises from the roots into the trunk on its journey upward as the sun rises. This phenomenon tells us that the most powerful time to absorb tree energy is at dawn and dusk. This then gives us a map or program for practice. To derive the most energy from trees stand on the south side at dawn or dusk!

TREE PRACTICE: FOLLOWING THE SUN

1. The south side of the tree is the most rich in energy. If we desire to receive the tree's life-giving energy, we need to approach the tree and stand facing the south side of the tree. This would mean that we face north.
2. The east side of the tree is most powerful in the AM hours.
3. The west side of the tree is useful when the practitioner wants to reduce excess energy.
4. When possible, start your Tree practice at dawn or dusk.
5. When activating energy with Tree practice, use the appropriate side of the tree to receive this energy.

These special times and compass directions are the ideal, but it should be noted that the tall giants of the forest can give us energy at

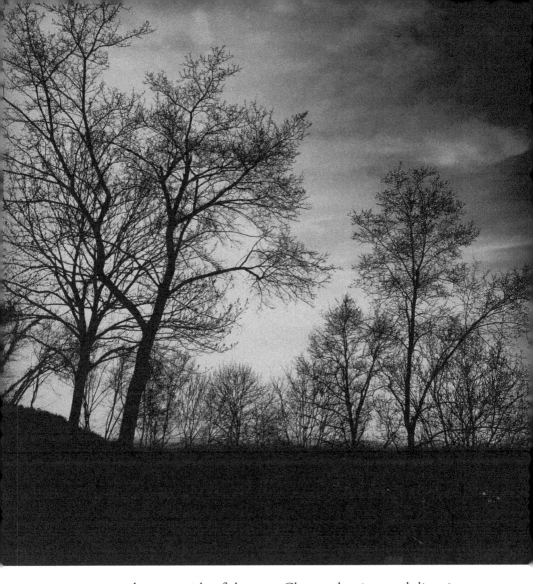

any time and on any side of the tree. Choose the time and direction that is most convenient for you. Remember, each time you practice, you gain sensitivity to tree energy and you start to feel the benefits getting stronger, more discernable.

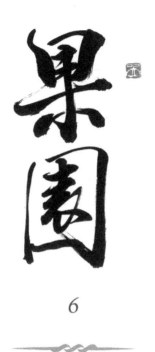

6

THE FIVE-ELEMENT ORCHARD

Perhaps there is no greater discipline, practice, or body of knowledge that encompasses the varied and rich aspects of Chinese thought than Traditional Chinese Medicine. It has a long and detailed history dating back 2500 years or more. If we begin to look at how Chinese Traditional Medical doctors see the human body and the universe, we can start to understand how this aspect of our environment (Trees) can become a power source of energy and a healing modality. According to the basic canon of Traditional Chinese Medicine (TCM), the root cause of almost all disease is a fundamental imbalance in yin/yang polarity in the body, and a lack of strong energy circulation.

YIN AND YANG

Yin and Yang are Taoist concepts that have become a way of seeing all of reality as being composed of two interdependent, yet opposing forces. The term Yin applies to the force in nature that is often described with the following adjectives: feminine, gentle, night, retreating, cool, soft. Yin could be said to be the pause between notes on a piano, as well as the withdrawal of the warrior's arm in preparation for attack. It is the coolness of the evening. Whereas, Yang adjectives include forceful, strength, projection, male, attacking, hot, hard. Yang is the strength in the male tenor's voice, as well as the force of a gale wind. It is the heat of the sun, as well as the warrior's attack.

Nature is in a constant motion of opposing forces, and when these go out of balance, the result is disharmony. This is true of our environment, as well as our bodies. But it is important to understand that the terms Yin and Yang really only exist in relation to their opposite. For example, the number 5 is yin to the yang of the number 10. Likewise, the same number 5 is Yang to the Yin of number 3. These Taoist concepts are relative to each other, not necessarily opposite. The key is balance. This is true for every aspect of body and mind, including every organ and every system of our metabolism. When these opposing forces go out of balance, illness is imminent. This basic polarity of yin and yang is the foundation of all existence and is the basis of all movement and change. And each aspect of existence and nature constantly seeks balance.

Yin and Yang are like two sides of a ball. One side is Yin, the other side is Yang. As you rotate the ball, you will see less of one side and more of the other. The duality is not separate but relative. If we consider something as either hot or cold, we could say that cold is the absence of hot (one is relative to the other). You can also have any combination of hot & cold to produce, warm, cool, luke warm etc.

One way of insuring or promoting this balance is to entrain with a like force. For this the TCM doctor or Qigong practitioner often go to an outside force of nature. The inner power of trees has been used since ancient times to help achieve this Yin and Yang balance. If we can connect to this inner energy and bring it into our system, the body will respond.

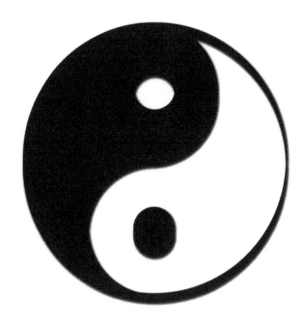

Yin Yang Symbol

ENERGY CIRCULATION

Qi or internal energy is in all things alive. Just as our circulatory system of blood running through veins and arteries, internal energy moves through the system through channels called meridians. When this energy is stopped, clogged, or absent in one of these channels, that part of the system to which the meridian line connects begins to suffer. It is interesting to note here that normal meridian lines usually begin in one of the extremities (hand or feet) and end in one of the life organs such as the lungs, kidneys, liver, heart, or spleen. Thus if the pericardium meridian does not have sufficient pressure, the heart can be in trouble. Traditional Chinese Medical doctors tell us that almost all disease and discomfort can be traced back to this lack of free flowing energy. One way to insure that this energy is moving through the system in a healthy way is to create strong Qi pressure, and this is often the focus of Qigong masters. The idea is to generate enough Qi energy, most importantly in the lower abdominal area, so as to create an abundant supply or "bank" of Qi to allow for the continuous and strong flow through the meridians and thus to every part of the body. This is similar to powerful water pressure from a source that allows for strong movement of water through pipes. The water does not stagnate, and it flushes out foreign, stagnant or unwanted material.

Trees also have an energy circulating through their roots, trunk, branches, and leaves. When the energy stops moving in a limb or branch, this part of the tree dies. No energy, no life.

Trees are a powerful energy source that we can tap into according to the Masters. This new, fresh, alive tree energy will, in turn, invigorate, strengthen, and enliven our own system of energy.

THE FIVE ELEMENTS

Ancient Taoist cosmology says from Yin and Yang come the five elements in nature: metal, water, wood, fire, and earth. All life then is an expression and combination of these five elements. Each of the elements has seemingly endless associations and interactions. Metal, for example, represents energy that has solidified. Metal is associated with our breath, the lungs, and the emotions of courage and strength. Water represents energy that moves downward. It is associated with the ears and the kidneys, as well as tranquility and the winter season. Wood represents energy that is growing and expanding. It is associated with the liver and the emotion of kindness, as well as our vision and the spring season. The fire element represents energy that is active. It is associated with the heart and the emotion of love. The season of the fire element is summer. The earth element represents energy that is stable and centered. It is associated with our sense of taste and the emotion of feeling balance and evenness. The season of the earth element is late summer.

The Qigong practitioner works with these elements to create a greater sense of balance, thus stabilizing yin and yang in the body. By maintaining this natural equilibrium among the different expressions of each of the five elements, the functions of the internal organs are regulated, as well as their related tissues and emotions.

In his book, *The Way of the Five Elements*, John Kirkwood asks us to imagine five huge gongs in the universe, each sounding and vibrating a different sound. Imagine every element in the universe and nature as vibrating to one of those gongs. Every aspect of nature, each organ, each part of the human physiology, each tree, and so on, vibrates and seeks balance or appropriate vibration. (7)

However, The Five Element theory and practice also extends to a myriad of expressions such as the season of the year, time of day, sounds, colors, etc., (See Five Element chart in appendix). Kirkwood further points out that stimulation of one element will affect and help to balance all other things that resonate with that element. For example, if the practitioner wanted to work with the emotion of fear, they could work with the energy in the kidneys, using those techniques associated with the water element such as Qigong exercises that work to gently expand and contract the kidneys. However, this action can be greatly enhanced by using additional aspects associated with the water element such as the color dark blue, and the sound, "chewww," as well as by practicing in the winter season or facing north.

Kirkwood also gives us a unique way of understanding how the five elements help to entrain or balance one another. Imagine having 50 guitars in a room, he writes. If you pluck the E string of just one guitar, all the E strings will start to vibrate as well (7). In the same way, the practitioner works on one element and all things associated with that element will benefit. Using the previous example, working on our kidneys to affect the emotion of fear will also benefit the physical kidneys, as well as the ears, our hearing, and our sense of feeling grounded.

This process of working on the body and internal organs using five-element theory is the foundation of the concept of Taoist alchemy. We are changing lead to gold! Qigong provides the mechanism through which one can change stress to vitality, negative emotions to positive, and scattered, ruminating thoughts to wisdom.

The ancient Masters also knew that trees partner with this mechanism of change. The power in a tree can be a potent ingredient that we add to the "cauldron" of the body to bring about this change.

Tree Fragrance

One of the great Taoist secrets is the fact that trees hold a powerful energy that can be used to bring about changes in all aspects of life—physical, emotional, and spiritual. Tree energy is very strong alchemic energy. The practitioner can open up to this energy, let it enter through one of "gates," and allow the system to "entrain" to the tree healing vibrations.

One of the pillars of Chinese Traditional Medicine is the use of herbal preparations, many of which come from the stems, bark, leaf, flower and fruit of trees. For these healers, the tree is a virtual pharmacy of healing treatments. However, there is one aspect of tree healing which is most potent—the tree's specific odor. Trees freely give off odors, which the ancient physicians learned were extremely powerful in healing a host of physical maladies and mental disturbances.

Fragrance or smell is a vibration, and vibration is energy. This is why aromatherapy works. You can synchronize your personal vibration to the smell of a particular fragrance. Certain fragrances can calm us down, while other fragrances can stir up emotions. Aromatherapy can also be used as a tool to enhance meditation.

> …there is one aspect of tree healing, which is most potent—
> the tree's fragrance!

These enlightened, highly intuitive Masters not only discovered that tree odors were strong medicine, but they also found that different odors coming from different trees were beneficial to specific organs. Following Five Element theory, certain tree odors have a healing effect for those physical organs, sense organs, and related parts of the body that are of the same element. For example, they discovered that the odor of the common birch tree was beneficial to those aspects of the human anatomy associated with metal: the lungs, the large intestine, and the skin. In fact, because of the Five Element association, the birch tree odor can be used to mitigate the "heavy" emotions of anxiety, depression, feeling of loss, etc., as well. And this is just one fragrance out of hundreds. As such, a simple walk through the forest is a walk through nature's pharmacy.

TREE COLOR

The ancient Masters knew that color, although an extremely subtle vibration, has the ability to soothe and tonify organ function. For example, the color white is associated with the metal element and helps to heal and strengthen the lungs. The color green is associated with the wood element and helps liver functioning. Red is associated with the fire element and works to balance and tone the heart. Dark blue is associated with the water element and helps kidney function, and yellow is associated with the earth element and helps to balance the spleen.

It is extremely interesting to note that the color of a tree—either its bark, flower or fruit—aligns to the five element theory that associates specific colors to specific organs. For example, the common birch tree with its magnificent white bark helps the human lungs. It is the combination of tree odor, associated tree color, and tree Qi that works its magic on the human system.

What follows is the Five Element Orchard. Specific trees with their unique odors and colors are grouped according to one of the five elements. This allows the practitioner to know what kind of tree to choose for healing and energy of specific imbalances, physical and mental. With each kind of tree in the Five-Element Orchard, there is a different procedure for absorbing its fragrance and receiving its benefit.

THE FIVE-ELEMENT ORCHARD

White Birch Tree (Alternate Tree: Aspen)

The white birch tree is deciduous and comes in over 60 different species. These beautiful white trees can often be found near rivers and lakes. Western herbalists use the leaves of the birch tree, which contain a high amount of vitamin C, to make medicine for urinary tract infections and maintaining kidney health. The medicinal properties of birch leaves are also used for correcting bladder, ureter, and urethra health infections. The sap of the birch tree contains sugar and proteins and is reported to have amazing healing properties. In short the Western herbalist uses the bark, leaves, and sap to heal everything from minor infections to cancer.

The ancient Taoist healers, however, focused more on this tree's fragrance, a more subtle medicine, but highly beneficial. These master physicians used the birch fragrance for asthma, chronic bronchitis, lung disorders, sinus problems, and skin disorders. The white color of this tree associates it with the metal element, and in Five Element Theory, this would connect it to the Lungs.

In addition to the physical healing properties of this tree's fragrance is the effective treatment of emotional concerns. The subtleness of the tree's odor allows it to be a healing agent for the refined emotional vibrations. In this regard, the Taoists would use the fragrance of the birch tree for those suffering from unresolved emotions, grief, or low self-esteem.

Unlike the tree's bark, leaves, and sap, this kind of healing involves an active role on the patient's part. The patient must make an

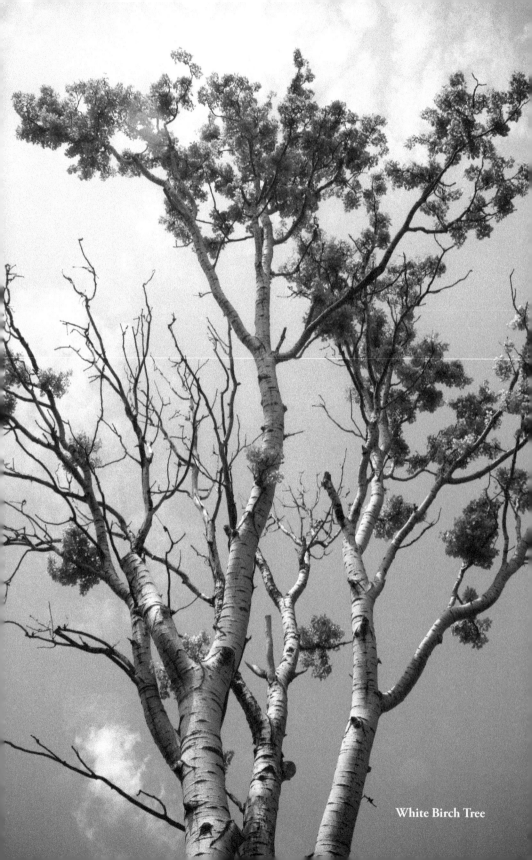

White Birch Tree

active effort to find the correct tree, and then use their knowledge of how to absorb this tree energy into their system. This form of healing does not involve taking a pill, eating bark, or ingesting sap. It is an active, self-healing exercise, and this can make a difference in the healing process, say the Masters.

Absorbing Birch Tree Fragrance

1. Approach your chosen birch tree and observe the long slender trunks with white bark and intermittent spots of dark. Birch trees are rarely alone. Feel welcomed into the family of beautiful white trees.
2. Stand in the Wuji stance for a moment to let you and the tree become accustomed to each other. Slowly raise your arms up as if to hug the tree, but keep the hands about two inches from actually touching the tree. As you do this, feel that your arms and hands have energetic extensions that go out and hold the tree trunk. The palms should face each other with the trunk in-between.
3. Hold this position and breathe deeply into the abdomen. Feel as if you are ingesting the tree's fragrance into your system
4. Feel the whiteness of the birch fill up your lungs, pushing out depression, anxiety, and feelings of loss. Let your lungs fill up with pure white light—the white of courage and strength.
5. Thank your tree for its energy and power and healing fragrance.

The Black Cypress (Alternate Tree: Pine Tree)

Black Cypress or Black Cypress Pine is often considered a native tree of Australia, but can be found throughout the world. This tree can be found along the Atlantic and Gulf coastal region in the US.

It is part of the conifer family and mostly valued for its timber and resin. It is a deciduous tree that loves water. Perhaps this is why it is associated with the water element in Five Element Theory. Although the tree itself is not considered a medicinal plant in terms of its bark, leaves, or sap, there is high praise for cypress oil. This part of the tree is said to help a host of medical concerns, including respiratory problems, arthritis, fungal infections and varicose veins.

The fragrance of the black cypress is perhaps the most powerful medicinal aspect of this beautiful tree. Because of its color and healing properties, the black cypress falls to the water element in Five Element Theory. This means that its special, fragrant odor is especially helpful for the kidneys. Actively absorbing the fragrance of this tree will help treat kidney disease, adrenal exhaustion, as well as low back pain.

In terms of emotional balance, the fragrance of the black cypress can help with fear and fear related concerns such as phobias, panic and anxiety attacks.

Absorbing Black Cypress Fragrance

1. Cypress trees are often found in swampy areas, near or in water. If possible approach your tree by water, preferably in a boat. Anchor your raft or canoe next to your chosen cypress. Feel the buoyancy and unsteady water beneath you.

2. Hold your hands out to the tree while you are standing facing away from the tree and your arms and hands stretched back so that your palms reach the trunk. Be sure you have steady footing before you do this. Ask your tree for anchorage in your life. Breathe in the fragrance of these giants and feel their strength and durability come into you. Feel this energy gather in the kidneys at your low back. Feel that this fragrance strengthens your kidney area, which becomes your anchor, your internal battery.

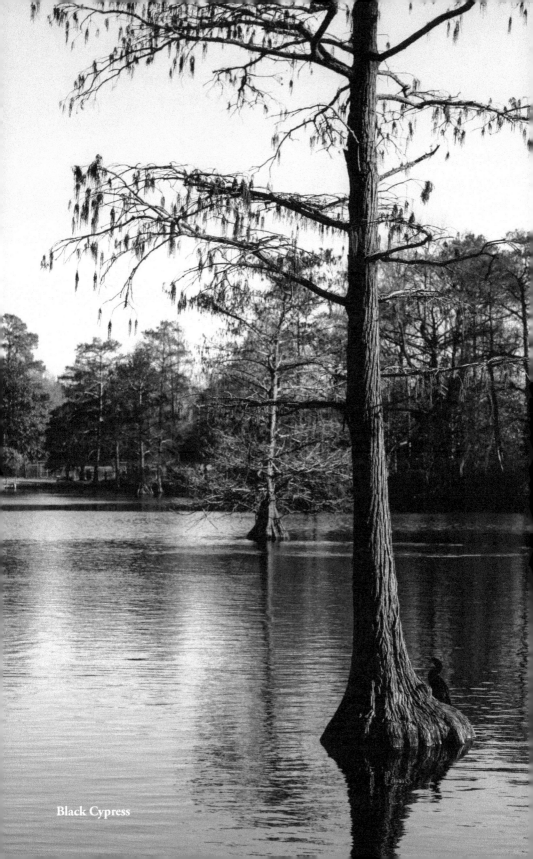

Black Cypress

3. Lower your arms down and stand quietly. Again feel or imagine the water underneath you, and feel the added strength of the cypress energy allowing you to be anchored, free of fear and trepidation.

4. Note that the Black Cypress tree is not found throughout the United States. The Pine tree is an excellent alternative. What organ and / or concern you want this tree to work for, will simply depend on your attention and intention.

The Pine Tree

The tree that has the attention of the ancient medical physicians and contemporary healers more than any other is the common pine tree. It is of the conifer family of which there are over 170 different species. It is found throughout the northern hemisphere, but is also found in less variety in southern climates. So powerful is this tree that every part of it has been used for one medicinal purpose or another—cones, bark, resin, sap, oil and needles. In fact, the needles are often made into a tea that is considered highly nutritional. Pine nuts are edible and full of nutrients that are important to digestion. This powerful tree has a host of beneficial properties, including the ability to improve circulation, protect against pathogens from outside the body, improve vision and boost immunity.

The early Taoists considered the pine tree, and its varieties, as holding the most energy. Perhaps this is why it holds its green throughout the winter. It is considered highly beneficial to practice Tai Chi and Qigong under or near pine trees. The shade is abundant and the soft needles provide a soft ground layer. Many aspects of the pine tree are found in Chinese Herbal compounds, as they are in the healing toolbox of Western herbalists. However, the one prevalent aspect of the pine tree that is often overlooked is the one so prevalent as you enter the pine forest—the wonderful pine fragrance. It is this tree odor that these Masters held in such high esteem.

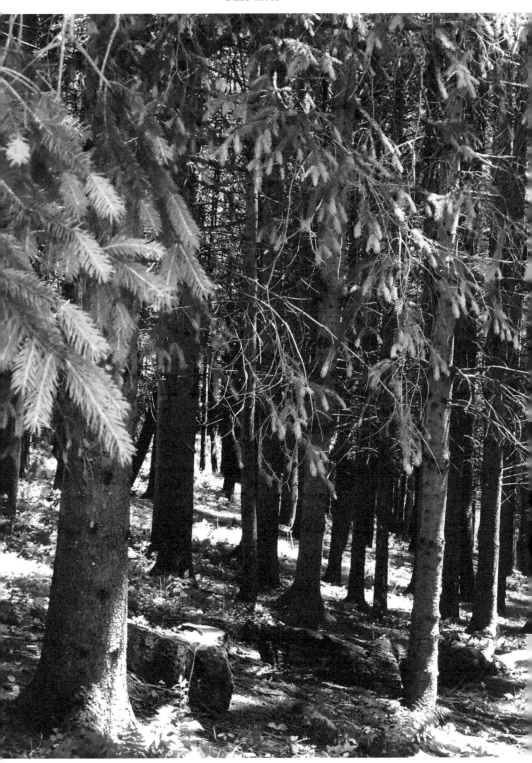

Due to its evergreen color and particular fragrance, the pine tree is beneficial to those elements of nature that are ruled by the wood element, which includes the liver and liver functioning. Disorders, which often fall in the wood element category, include headache and migraines, joint pain, arthritis, hormonal imbalances and high blood pressure. In terms of emotional imbalance, improper liver function is responsible for anger, frustration, and volatile emotions. When we suffer from one or more of these imbalances, one can seek refuge under the power of the pine tree—especially the pine fragrance.

Once when I was studying with my Master, Shifu Jiang Jian-ye, in Albany, NY, the topic of the lesson turned to training outside. Literally millions of Tai Chi, Qigong, and Martial artists train outside in the parks in China in the morning. At times, in some cities, the parks are so filled with practitioners in the morning, that one has to get up especially early to get space to practice. So adamant and strong in their practice, some enthusiasts go out into exceptionally bad air quality with facemasks to practice their Tai Chi.

Shifu explained the value of outside air and inside air. In most cases the air outside is fresher, filled with negative ions, especially in the morning. "Is it good to practice in a forest then, Shifu?" one student asked.

"Yes," he replied, "and if you can find a pine tree, that is best."

Pine trees, Shifu explained, are the type of tree with the strongest Qi. Perhaps this is why they hold their green color in winter. When asked what else might the practitioner look for in choosing the very best outdoor practice area, Shifu responded by encouraging practitioners to be near a large body of water, if you can find it. "And face east," he added.

It wasn't until some years later, when I was living in Iowa for a short time period, did I find the ideal training ground outside. One of my students said that after each class, he would go to Waterworks Park a few miles away, to practice what he had learned. It was a nice day, so I decided to take my whole class to the park. We immediately found a grove of pine trees with a large flat surface area for training. I looked up and saw the lake, not 20 yards away. I had to ask, "What direction are we facing?"

"East" was the reply. We had found our ideal spot.

Procedure for absorbing Pine Tree Fragrance

1. Approach your chosen pine tree or conifer. Observe its height, feel the pine needles beneath your feet, and feel the coolness beneath the canopy.
2. Sit down on the soft needles at the base of the tree and begin to feel as if you are taking a complete energetic Pine bath. Again, feel the soft needles; allow the tree's aura to surround you.
3. Let the darkness of the pine and its neighbors bring you into a wonderful Pine world—a Pine Palace of aroma, softness, and cooling energy. Pay close attention to each sense and then focus on the pine fragrance. See it as cooling green energy that you are ingesting into your system. Let it fill up your whole body. Imagine or feel that there is no difference between your inner body and the aura of the tree. Be in it and of it as you sit quietly for a few moments.

The Apple Tree (Alternate Tree: Red Maple)

The apple tree is actually of the rose family and is deciduous. This is a tree that is cultivated worldwide with as many as 7,500 varieties, with the Red Delicious being the most common. You will find apple trees in both northern and southern hemispheres. The fruit of the apple tree has been linked to health for centuries.

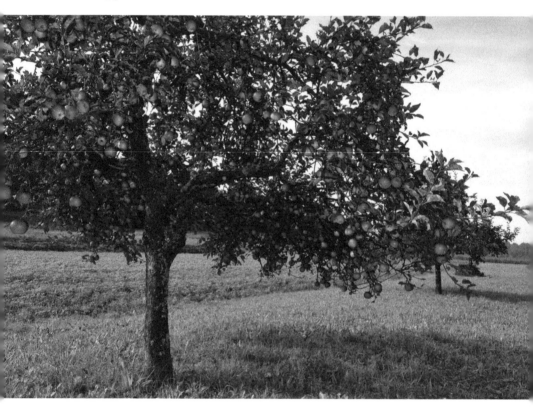

Apple Tree

Western health professionals have long talked about the common apple as rich in fiber and an aid to digestion and the colon, as well as good for treating anemia and helping to control diabetes.

Traditional Chinese Medical professionals have other uses for the common apple, including the support of lung function, skin rejuvenation, and help for asthma sufferers. They also use apples, sometimes in preparation with other fruit and herbs, to strengthen the intestines, stop diarrhea and constipation, as well as strengthen the heart.

These benefits are a boon to mankind and could even be called miraculous. However, when we learn how to absorb the apple tree's fragrance, we open a pathway to a wonderful host of other healing properties—emotional and physical.

The apple tree gives us access to the fire element, as suggested by its red color of the fruit (green and yellow varieties still fall into the fire element category). The fragrance of the apple tree was used by the ancient Masters to mitigate a large group of abnormalities such as heart disease, heart palpitations, mouth sores, insomnia, acid reflux, and poor memory. On an emotional level the fragrance of the apple tree works on an inability to love, irritability, hastiness, and feeling of a broken heart.

Tree Fragrance—Procedure for absorbing energy from the apple tree

1. Approach your chosen apple tree. Observe its beauty and bounty. Stand roughly two to three feet away from the trunk. Stand in the Wuji stance and slowly raise the arms up high over your head with the palms on either side of the trunk of your chosen tree.
2. Make your breath long, slow, and deep. On each in-breath take in the odor of the tree and feel that it is coming through your palms, down the arms and into the heart.
3. Now place the two middle fingers of each hand on the center of your chest (acupoint CV17 "The Sea of Tranquility) and put your full attention on your heart. Imagine that the fragrance has not only entered your heart, but has also purified each chamber holding old feelings or emotions. Let the fragrance have a red

color and feel it in, around, throughout the heart place. Do this for an additional few minutes. Drop your hands down to your sides. Thank your tree, thank your heart.

The Willow Tree

The willow tree is also called sallows and osiers. It is deciduous with over 400 species. It is found mostly in temperate regions of the northern hemisphere. It has an interesting, if not mysterious, history. Japanese folklore tells us that the willow trees are ghosts, while English legend talks of willow trees as sinister and capable of uprooting themselves for nefarious purposes.

However, Western herbalists and botanists have long touted the willow tree's benefits, which include its anti-inflammatory properties and benefits to arthritis sufferers. Willow trees are also said to ease menstrual cramps, soothe stomach disorders and reduce fever.

The Traditional Chinese physicians are particularly interested in willow tree bark. It is used in TCM for fever, headache, pain, jaundice, venereal disease and inflammation. The Chinese Masters also use the willow tree's gum, long twigs, and seeds in their prescribed teas and herbal mixtures.

From the perspective of Five-Element Theory, the fragrance of the willow tree is particularly important to the earth element, and specifically the spleen organ. In terms of the physical body, an imbalance in the Earth Element is responsible for stomach issues, weight gain, diabetes, hypoglycemia, as well as nausea, overeating, and craving sweets. Stagnant or abnormal energy in the spleen will also cause certain emotions to arise, specifically, worrying, obsessive thoughts, feelings of martyrdom and ambivalence.

Absorbing the fragrance of the willow tree

1. The spring time is the best time to look for your willow tree,

and if you can find one that grows near a body of water, all the better. Approach your chosen tree with softness and reverence. Ask the tree's permission to work with you. The willow tree is a beautiful lady, and her long flowing hair is particularly inviting. The willow tree's strands of yellow often reach the ground.

2. See if you can go inside this canopy and feel as if she has embraced you. Let your arms hang at your sides as you stand in Wuji fashion. Feel as if your arms are but two more string-like branches of the willow.

3. Breathe in the fragrance of the tree with long, slow breaths. Do this 36 times.

4. Once you feel that your body has absorbed the willow fragrance fully, imagine you have roots from the bottom of your feet sinking deep into the earth. Feel earth energy. As you inhale, bring this cool, willow root energy up into your body through your spinal cord. When you have reached the crown, exhale and imagine yellow light coming out of your crown and cascading out and down all over your body. Continue this breathing and color imagery for 9-12 breaths.

5. Come to rest for 2-3 minutes. Thank your willow, smile to your spleen. It will smile back.

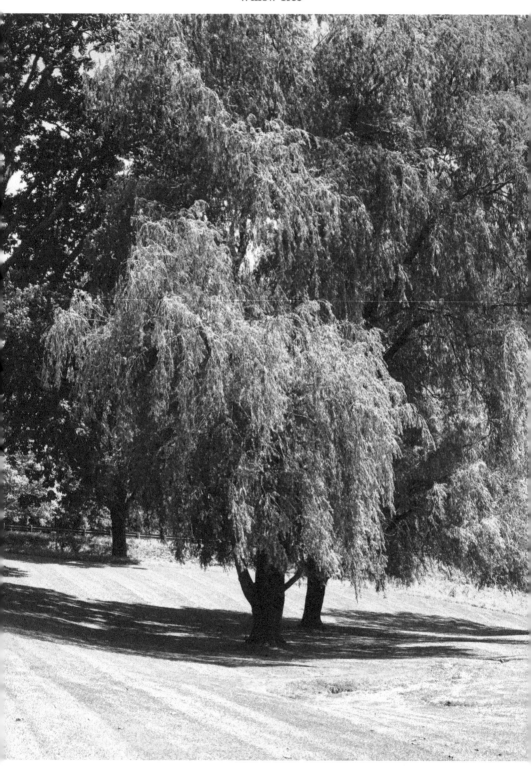

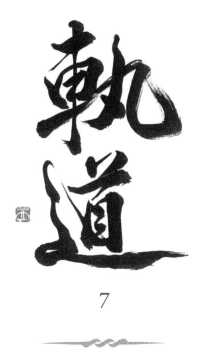

7

ORBITS OF ENERGY

A focal point of Chinese Traditional Medicine is Qi circulation. If fresh energy is moving through the system, stagnant or stale energy is flushed out. In order to promote this movement of Qi throughout the system, the Taoist Masters prescribed those Qigong techniques which provided the practitioner with strong "Qi Pressure." If there is a strong build-up of energy, especially in the Tan Tien (abdominal area), this pressure will ensure the free movement of Qi through the meridian lines that run throughout the body. If the pressure is strong, the flow of Qi is strong, and this means little or no stagnation, which means no disease.

The early Masters also developed another procedure for Qi circulation called the Microcosmic Orbit, sometimes called "Small Circulation." It was also known as the "Self Winding Wheel." This procedure is a method of creating an orbit of energy in the system, which bathes the entire body. There are numerous variations, but almost all of them combine breathing, visualization, and sensing energy. The pathways for this orbit involve two main channels in the body: the Du meridian that runs up the back of the body, and the Ren meridian, which runs down the front. By consciously moving energy through these two main channels, the smaller meridian lines are fed with energy, which is then carried to the organs, limbs, etc. The practice of microcosmic orbit is usually done in a sitting posture, but it can also be done in one of several standing postures called Zhan Zhuang.

The Microcosmic Orbit is important, as it is at the heart of many Taoist Qigong practices and is considered an important technique for overall health and longevity. Like the concept of three energies (Heaven, Earth, and Man), the Orbit practice has its roots in the *I Ching*, the classic Taoist text of the twelfth Century BCE. Later Taoists such as Lao Tzu and Chuang Tzu referred to it as an important practice to move energy through the subtle channels.

THE ENERGY ORBIT OF TREES

We have already spoken about how trees reach to the sun during the day and seek nutrients from the soil at night, that there is a natural movement of energy from the canopy to the roots and the reverse as the day begins. This is a natural flow of energy in nature and is similar to the Orbit we create in our own bodies. And yet trees move this energy without the help of movement, exercise, or cognitive incentive. It is a powerful energetic force of movement that happens constantly and silently. The early Taoists knew the power of tree energy and sought to "tap in" to this cycle.

A COMBINATION OF ORBITS

Can we combine the human Microcosmic Orbit with the Tree Energy Orbit in order to absorb, at least in part, the Tree's energy? It turns out that the procedure to accomplish this is relatively simple. We stand near our chosen tree at the edge of the outermost reach of the tree's canopy. In most cases, we are then standing on top of the most outward spread of the root system. From here it is a matter of tuning into the energy orbit of the tree as well as your own. The practitioner feels the energy of the tree's roots as it moves up through the trunk to the canopy and back down. Because the practitioner stands at the edge of the canopy, she can include her orbit in the loop.

Important Points

1. Each tree in the forest has a circuit of energy that runs from the canopy to the root system and back.
2. Humans have a similar orbit of energy running through two major energy channels: the Ren and Du channels in the front and back of the trunk of the body respectively.
3. The practitioner can blend these two channels together to form a giant Tree loop, thus allowing the practitioner to "tap" into the tree energy.

The Microcosmic Orbit and Tree Orbit Combined

1. Decide on the tree with which you wish to work. Look for one that has a relatively wide canopy that extends out from the trunk.
2. Stand at the edge of the canopy so that your head is right under the furthest point of the canopy spread.
3. Begin by practicing the Microcosmic orbit. As you breathe in, feel a sense of energy go up your back through the Du or Governing meridian, one of eight extraordinary channels. The Du meridian runs from the bottom of your spine, up the back and over the head. Then, as you exhale, imagine that

energy is moving down the front channel called the Ren or Conception channel, which runs from the your tongue level to the perineum. Breathe in this pattern for a few minutes to feel your own energy loop through your system. (Keep the tongue on the roof of the mouth during this practice).

4. Once you have created this strong circuit, you will include the tree's own orbit into yours.

5. Start by putting your attention on the very top of the tree's canopy. Imagine and sense energy going down through the trunk of the tree into the root system. Tune into the sense of strong earth energy as you allow it to come up into your feet through the acupoint Kidney 1, that is located at the bottom of the foot, in the center.

6. Next feel this earth/tree energy loop into your orbit by bringing it up into the Du meridian along the back of your spine and over the top of the head. Continue following the energy as it travels to come down the Ren meridian in front up the Du meridian.

7. On this second loop, once the energy reaches the head or crown point, direct it up the canopy of the tree to the very top. Repeat steps 5-7.

8. This completes one whole circuit of combined tree and human energy orbits. Continue this energy pattern for a few minutes or longer. Each time you loop the tree's orbit and your orbit, you will start to feel a stronger sense of the power of tree energy moving through you.

9. When you want to end the orbit practice, feel the energy enter your body for the last time and settle into the low abdomen. Rotate your hands clockwise on this area to allow the energy to store in the abdomen, the area the Masters called the "Elixir Field."

(Please note: This explanation of the Microcosmic Orbit is cursory, as

whole books have been written about this process. Although the process is simple as explained, the reader might want to learn more about the Orbit practice from a teacher or do a more in-depth study before working with a tree's orbit.)

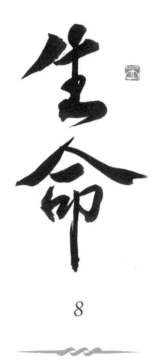

8

LIFE BLOOD OF THE TREE

In terms of learning how to absorb energy from trees, one needs to understand that trees are living, breathing entities with their own special nervous systems and energy lines. If we tap into their energy system, we exchange energy with them, and this reciprocity gives us a new, pure nature Qi. This harmonizes and balances our own bodies, and we walk out of the forest more refreshed, clear, and energized. In fact, tree Qi may add an energy element that you are missing. We all have energy deficiencies and tree energy may fill that gap.

Tree energy has the ability to calm the mind. Observe a giant Oak tree. Observe its stillness, steadiness, and rootedness. That tree's energy carries those qualities. That energy is a gift to you, as your exhaled carbon dioxide is a gift to it.

The early Masters are said to have gone to the forest to calm and still the mind. Years of meditation and Qigong practice among the trees elevated their Shen or spirit, and they found not only connection to the trees, but to all of nature.

In our modern lives we cannot escape to live for years in the forest among the trees. However, we can periodically make a tree connection, but we must make the effort to set the process up.

With this following tree practice, it is recommended that you work with the tree at night. Working with trees during the day can be useful if working on tumors or muscle and tendon problems, but the cultivation process of absorbing tree energy is best done after sunset according to Master David Verdesi.

TREE POWER

Start by standing near your tree of choice in Wuji, a stance that lines up your body to allow energy to flow effortlessly through the meridians. Have both your feet perfectly flat to the ground. Soften your knees, tuck in the sacrum slightly, spread your scapulae and slightly round your shoulders. Keep your chin in so that the crown of the head is facing directly towards the heavens. This "Wuji" stance is optimized in complete stillness.

Stand facing the tree about one arm-length away, palms facing directly towards the tree. Move the palms up and down the trunk and try to feel a connection to the energy within the tree as you mentally go inside the tree.

Start by moving the **energy of the tree** up and down a short distance, gradually lifting the energy further and further up. Eventually imagine you are moving a geyser of energy up to the peak of the canopy and then pulling it down to the ground. You are moving the "blood" of the tree.

At this point you are learning to experience moving energy outside of yourself as well. You are shifting the energy all around you. This will strengthen your Qi.

As the hands come down the tree, bend the knees slightly. Sense the movement of Qi in your body and the Qi of the tree at the same time. Moving tree energy up and down, align your own energy with the same up and down movement. The synchronization of tree and human energies will start to blend. You are literally connecting to Mother Nature on a most profound level. On an inner, subtle level, you and that tree are one.

Do this movement as your intuition dictates. Then slow the movement down and go back to the Wuji pose for a short time. Meditate with your giant, bark-covered friend. Feel the kinship.

Learning to move and synchronize with tree energy can become not only a wonderful Qi cleansing activity, but it can also serve as a link to our connection to nature. This is a movement towards en-lightenment. We slowly begin to loosen our confining attachment to this body, this mind, and we begin to explore how we are connected to all of nature, all of life.

An extremely accomplished Qigong and Tibetian Buddhist Master, David Verdesi has been practicing internal arts since he was fourteen years old. He has traveled extensively throughout, China, Russia, Tibet and Mongolia., constantly seeking Masters with the truest, most power-ful teachings. Researching and comparing his own experiences with those of mystics, yogis, cave dwellers, saints and genuine enlightened beings, Master Verdesi is an extremely accomplished energy practitioner. His mastery now reaches into the forest.

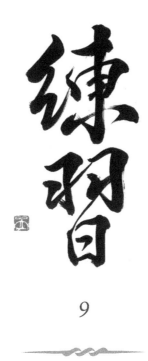

9

PUTTING IT ALL TOGETHER

The tree energy practices in this book are the culmination of the work of a number of contemporary Qigong Masters, as well as the ancient Masters, who first taught us the power, majesty, and benefit of working with these tall forest beings. Consequently, each practice can be done independent of the other. With a sense of openness, approach each one of these practices with the spirit of experimentation. Which ones feel energizing, calming, or healing? You may find a practice that, more than all the others, works for you and your sense of Qi.

Or you may want to combine techniques. Here are a few scenarios to try:

1. Find the tree with which you wish to work. Decide on an appropriate stance to take for the part of the body or organ on which you want to work. For example, find a tree and adopt

the "Hands up high" stance for your heart—either to work on the physical heart or the emotions associated with the heart such as greater love and openness. In this stance, with attention on the heart, practice the microcosmic orbit with the tree's orbit. (Chapter7). Allow the smell of the tree and the energy of the tree to move through your system.

2. Find the kind of tree that is conducive to the particular organ you want to work on. For example, choose an apple tree to work on the heart. Approach the tree and stand on the south side of the tree facing north. Sense and feel the energy of the tree and adopt a restful standing pose. Feel that energy enter your heart. Smile to the heart.

3. Follow the sun. Stand facing the side of your chosen tree that faces the sun. In the morning, face the east side of your tree. During the late morning to late afternoon, face the south side of the tree. And face the west side of the tree during the setting sun (this would be appropriate if you wished to reduce excitement or an overly active mind).

4. What is your intent? Using trees to generate more energy may be your focus. Start by working with Qi stances (Chapter 4). If your idea is to heal a particular part of the body or emotion, the Five Element Orchard (Chapter 6) may be a place to visit. If you wish to have a more spiritual experience, Life Blood of the Tree (Chapter 8) may be a great help.

5. Combine the practices in Chapter 4 with the techniques of Chapter 6. Each practice has a different way of harvesting tree energy. Combine and play with it. See which way feels best to you. Put these practices into your "toolbox," so to speak, and pull out what your intuition says is best for a particular tree, time of day, or emotion that you are feeling. And perhaps the most significant practice is this: master your tree practice technique, enter the forest with impartiality and openness and let the tree's own wisdom find you and show you the way. Good luck!

THE FIVE ELEMENT ORCHARD

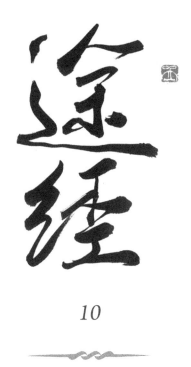

10

FIELDS BEYOND THE ORCHARD—TREE BREAKS

Now that you've learned to find trees that can balance your body and emotions and how to harvest energy from them, you can use any of the following special techniques to deepen your experience in the forest.

Entering the Present—Loop Trail

While walking in a forest, choose a wooded path that loops back to your starting point. Most loops could be said to be "lazy circles," and your journey should be in a circle. You should not pass any point twice, each turn will be a fresh experience, a new discovery, as in a Chinese Cup Garden, where every turn is a moment of discovery and transcendence. Your loop trail will allow you to travel, not as a journey from point A to point B, but in a manner that feels more "whole," or complete. So often we go through life thinking about the future or remembering the past. Your trail will take you away from the feeling of going from here to there, and pull you into the experience at hand—the now!

Entering the Present—Heart Breath

Move your breath to the heart place and imagine you can breathe from this area. This allows you get in touch with the body, and you can begin to see the beauty around you with your skin as well as your eyes. Keep breathing into the heart and shift your awareness to the body—drop into the present moment and be here with this forest rich with life. You are part of it.

Have a Chat with Mother Nature

Walking down the wooded path, along the waterfront, or through the park has proven scientific benefits on many levels. As you walk, can you have the feeling that you are not alone? Do you feel the presence, the personality of each tree, mountain ridge, or lake that you see? Bring this feeling into reality by chatting with nature. In whispered breath tell each tree how you feel. Are you grateful, charmed, comforted? Express your gratitude for the beauty, mystery, and joy of each element you pass. The oak tree that you see will patiently listen and perhaps respond in its own silent way.

Smile to the Beauty of the Woods

A traditional Chinese Cup garden is usually designed around a lake or small body of water, which is surrounded by nature. The garden masters would use flowers, blossoming trees, small water falls, and rolling landscapes around the lake so to create stunning beautiful vistas at every turn. The idea was to create such breathtaking picturesque views at every turn, so as to allow the sojourner to transcend the limits of time and space and be part of nature's fullness.

While walking in the forest, lakeside, or park, pause and smile to the transcendent beauty of the trees, water, and landscape. Does nature smile back? Go and see.

Auras and Webs

Walking deeper into the forest, notice a coolness and silence—as if the trees themselves were fanning a quiet soft breeze. Trees, like all things alive, project an energy or aura. This energy field around us humans is called the Wei Chi. Around trees it can extend many feet from its trunk and canopy. Like humans, trees use this aura to protect, balance, and center. It is the life of the tree that is bigger than the tree.

As you walk through the forest, you pass through their energy. In fact, you pass through layer on top of layer of tree aura energy, that forms a dense web. As you continue to breath softly in your present moment awareness, you can begin to feel this web as cooling, life affirming, comforting.

Move your gaze up the canopy of any large tree that draws your attention, to one that rises above its forest neighbors. Look at the crown of the canopy against the sky. Look with "soft eyes" and notice the subtle, but distinct light emanating from the treetop and the rest of the sky. This is the aura of the tree, often extending beyond the canopy two or three feet. It is a glow of light, the inner energy of the tree that extends out. This tree aura practice is also a good way to train your eye to see auras of humans. With practice you might see distinct colors and shades. Let the tree be your training.

Shades of Green

Find a spot where the land gently slopes down, allowing you to see the top of the forest spread out before you. Look out over the expanse of nature and begin to count how many different shades of green you can see—those near you, as well as the ones on the distant ridge. Notice that this practice allows you to focus gently on nature in this moment. Counting the shades of green brings you to the present moment—an incredibly easy mental task that happens now. Do this for a few moments. How many did you count? Too many to count?

Nature Moves

Observe the beautiful landscape and notice the movements. Everywhere nature is gently moving: wind across the grasses, shimmering leaves, tree boughs gently lifting, the sway of willows, shaking aspen leaves. Find a natural movement, something specific. Fix your attention on it and keep it there. Try to avoid the mind drifting into thoughts. Notice that as you do this, you begin to settle down on the inside, your heart begins to beat slower, and you feel settled. Let the movement of nature bring you to stillness.

Especially in Western culture, we tend to sit too much—at home on the couch, at work at our desk, or in the car. And yet when we do move, it can be rather erratic, quick, jerky as we dart here and there, always changing direction. While observing nature's slow, gentle, flowing movements, our own internal energy or Qi also begins to flow, and we begin to develop a stronger affinity with the power around us. The violin of the soul begins to tune to the orchestra of nature.

Soar with the Birds

Turn your gaze upward and search the sky. Find a bird, perhaps a large bird of prey—hawk, eagle, osprey. Let go of your feeling of looking awkward and extend your arms out to your sides. Mimic your friend high in the sky. Mirror the wing patterns of your bird with your arms. Be free, float, and dance. Keep your eye on your bird. Feel the freedom of flight and glide on the wind with effortlessness, ease, and joy. Come down to earth, feel rooted again to Mother Earth, and breathe.

This technique is a very freeing experience. For a brief moment we drop our inhibitions of how to act, and we play—as we did as children. Who has not looked to the sky and wished for the freedom of flight?

Let the Tree Hug You

The term "Tree Hugger" has supporters, as well as detractors. Have you given thought to allowing the tree to hug you?

Stand on the edge of the tree's canopy. Observe its magnificent color and allow the green of the leaves to embrace you, touching your skin, and then penetrating each pore and cell. Feel the whole body cloaked in green. Now approach your tree and put your arms around it, as a warm thank you.

Listening to Distance

Sound, especially distant sounds, can be a doorway to another world, a world of infinite space and silence. And often it is the most distant sound that awakens the deepest part of our soul. If the sound is intermittent, such as successive cries of the hawk, or a foghorn out to sea or the distant train whistle, pay attention to the silence in-between.

Using our sense of hearing is a wonderful way to connect to trees and nature. During your walk in the forest, park or lakeside, stand still and listen. Just listen. Allow the silence of the tree to embrace you. Now listen more carefully. Take note of the most subtle sounds: the gentle wind in the trees, the clicking of branches, the scurry of squirrels. Now close your eyes and identify the most distant sound you hear. Take notice of the space between you and that sound. Allow your consciousness to expand and feel that space as part of you. Are you not connected to all of nature?

Aromas

Find a pine grove. Feel the needles beneath your feet and how the ground softens and feels so different. Take a deep breath and absorb the aroma. Let it fill your lungs and reach deeper into the lower lobes of the lungs; let it fill the abdomen as the diaphragm gently lowers down with each breath. Now pick up a handful of pine needles and notice the pine aroma—different, even woodsier now. Pick a tree and smell the bark, and then notice the strong smell of sap. Now stand back and breathe in the aroma of the whole pine forest. Let this pine essence enter and heal you.

Pine Needle Walking

Find a grove of pine trees, remove your shoes, and quietly walk over the soft carpet of needles. Feel and notice your connection to Mother Earth. Be present at each step, feeling the pull of gravity gently hugging you to the planet. As you walk barefoot, take in the aroma of the pine and feel the intoxication of the scent fill every part of your body.

Now, if possible, circumambulate your pine friend in both clockwise and counterclockwise directions. Be quiet and still enough to notice how different each direction feels on the different parts of your body. The great masters of Bagua (an internal system of circles that is used in martial arts and energy building) in China claim that walking in a clockwise fashion will energize and wake-up the nervous system, and walking in a counterclockwise fashion will sedate and calm the nervous system. Because the simple circle does not have a destination, it is easy to use this technique to access and dwell in the present moment. Keep your attention on the tree in the center of your circle. Walking in both directions will feel balancing and grounding.

Forest Fresh

Bring attention to your breath and gently increase the length of your inhale and exhale, but do not do this to the point of discomfort. Feel the coolness of the forest on your nostrils with each inhale and feel the release of warm air as you breathe out. Continue this breathing as you walk for a few yards and then softly repeat mentally the two following words with each breath: Inhale saying "Forest" and then exhale saying "Fresh" to yourself. Continue as you breathe and walk, "Forest" / "Fresh." "Forest" / "Fresh" (6).

Now try the word "Earth" on the inhale and "Home" on the exhale. Which combination of words coordinated with your breathing in and out feels best to you? Remember to breathe deeply, comfortably, and continuously. You can coordinate the breathing with your steps and create a wonderful rhythm of body, breath, and mental image.

I first learned about this use of breath from the Vietnamese Zen Buddhist Master Thich Nhat Hanh. His writing extols the virtues of using the breath to come to silence. The breath becomes that doorway to the infinite. It is a beautiful practice.

Standing on Mother Earth.

Stand rooted on the earth and feel the earth beneath you. Feel the pull of gravity. Imagine you are standing on a huge rubber play ball, a ball we call Earth. Imagine that it is filled with air and thus very soft and giving. Gently bounce up and down, as if on this large rubber ball and feel the give of earth with each bounce. As you do this, bring your attention inside and feel internal organs, fascia, tendons, and muscles gently moving up and down with the give of each earth bounce. Now come to stillness.

In Qigong practice there are multiple ways to "bounce." In most cases bouncing the body is considered purification, as it gently breaks up any stagnation of energy and tightness due to stress, posture, or improper movement. The key in shaking or bouncing is to let go and completely relax the body to help facilitate the release of negative energy.

Touching

Find a the tree that attracts you. Approach your tree with reverence and gratitude. Place both palms on each side of the tree—feel the fullness of the trunk. Feel how steady it is, round, thick, and still. It is still but it is very alive. As you hold your tree, close your eyes and try to feel the life in the tree. Can you feel the tree breathing? Does it have a heartbeat? Go deep into it.

Now, pull the palms away, no more than an inch or two. Do you have the feeling that you are still holding the tree? Can you feel the aura, the energy coming off the trunk? Does that aura extend further out? Does it engulf you? Are you in the energetic embrace of this gentle giant? Now find another tree, a different kind of tree and shape perhaps.

Notice the difference. Are they not as different as we all are?

Heart to Heart Meditation

According to research done by the HearthMath Institute, the energy of the heart creates a dome shaped electromagnetic field around us in 360 degrees that radiates about 3 feet away from our body. This field is imprinted with our intentions and emotions and provides an unseen level of connection and communication with all living systems.

Here is a meditation that can foster a deeper sense of connection with a chosen tree and to all of nature.

1. Choose your tree, one that attracts you or "calls" you to it. Approach the tree with reverence, and ask its permission to do this practice.
2. Sit or stand in front of the tree. Bring your attention to your heart center in the center of the chest, and breathe into it. Feel or imagine that the breath is actually moving in and out through the heart center.
3. Stay with this breath for a couple of minutes until you feel calm and centered.
4. Begin to sense the "heart" or pulse of the tree. Feel or imagine the tree's heart pulsing in sync with your own.
5. Introduce a feeling of love, care, or gratitude into your heart centered breath
6. As you exhale love or gratitude, feel the tree inhaling this feeling into its heart. As the tree "exhales" feel yourself inhaling gratitude emanating from the tree's heart.
7. Continue this exchange of breath and love or gratitude with the tree for a few minutes, until you feel a deep connection or oneness with the tree.
8. After a few minutes, relax the breathing. Allow this gratitude or love to infuse every cell of your body and every cell of the tree.
9. Now let this blessing of gratitude fill the space around you, let it fill the entire forest. Send this blessing to the entire planet, and even into the space beyond the earth.
10. Then sit in spacious stillness with your tree, feeling your energy mingling with the energy of the universe.

Hugged by the Approaching Darkness

Walk into the forest at sunset. As the night slowly approaches, ask yourself if you feel as if you are being hugged by the engulfing darkness. Look to the west and see the gold and orange hues of the sun as this light plays in the trees. There is softness here, a stronger feeling of quiet. The forest is beginning to shift slowly into its night-time mode. Be aware of the changes: notice the cooler temperature on your skin, notice your conversations have become quieter, and notice how easy it has become to feel comfortable with the present moment.

In schools of mysticism, tenets of religions, and various occult traditions, the time of dusk is a magical time of the day. It is easier to perceive the unseen world and feel a sacred pause between activity and rest, similar to those delicate few moments just before falling asleep.

Star Food

Go into the forest or park at night. Stand quietly and look up into the splender of the night sky, especially when there is a clear view of the canopy of stars.

As you gaze up, use your right hand to make a scooping motion so as to gather the light of the stars. Channel the twinkling starlight into your crown. You are pulling in star food.

Feel that light come down into the spinal cord and spread throughout the body. Keep gathering starlight, let it fill your body. Now close the eyes and go within. Feel the indescribable expanse of the night sky within. You are the universe, you are starlight.

Stars Between the Branches

Many of us will remember the time when, as children, we would lie on the grass at night and look up at the stars, either at summer camp or in the back yard. Recall the wonder of the vastness of space and the billions of stars.

Find a comfortable place to lie down outside under the stars, but this time, if possible, lie beneath a large tree, perhaps an oak, chestnut, or apple tree. Gaze up at the branches and see the stars in the space between the branches. The experience can be one of awe, a feeling we have lost for so many years.

A Final Thought

A number of years ago I was visiting several of my young students in Saratoga Springs, NY. Late one afternoon I was invited to join them at a local teahouse, and, upon entering, something caught my eye. I surveyed the list of tea offerings on a chalkboard above the register, and it was the name of one of the teas that was to change the way I looked at trees and nature in general. The tea selection was called, "The Space Between the Branches"—I was immediately fascinated and enamored! Why was I drawn to something that was nothing? The image of empty space between oceans of green leaves was to become a doorway for me to experience the innermost beauty and sacredness of trees. I began to understand that trees could bring me to silence, and I realized how sacred the woods could become. Was this the same experience I had while sitting on the beach on Cape Cod, listening to the haunting foghorn drifting across the water? Was this the same experience I had had when hearing the commuter train whistle trail off, as I waited for my father to reach the station?

The lonely sound of the foghorn and the haunting sound of the train whistle were sacred to me. Do not sound and image at their most subtle levels share the same home? The space between the branches of the sycamore tree outside my window was nature at its most silent, mysterious, and bewitching best.

Trees now became more holy, and I lost interest in identifying them by leaf or bark or even naming them. These giant beings of the forest were now guardians of my inner peace, continuously meditating with immeasurable patience.

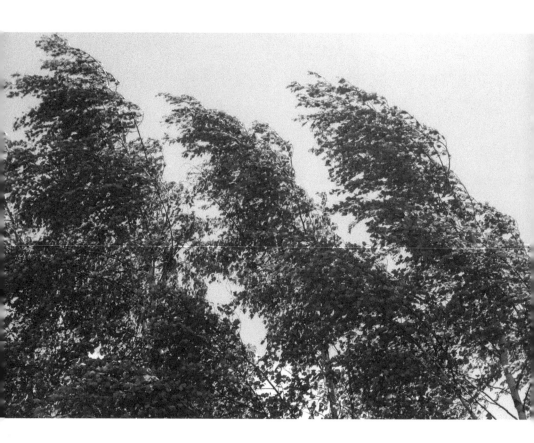

"The trees began to whisper
and the wind began to roll
And in the wild March morning
I heard them call my soul."
(Alfred Lord Tennyson
"The May Queen")

APPENDIXES

Appendix A

LIST OF TREE PRACTICES

Appendix B

~~~~~

ENERGY GATES

The early Taoists not only were able to map out how the energy or Qi moves through the body through passageways called meridians, but they also recognized that the body has a series of special pressure points that, when stimulated, can influence the flow of energy within their respective meridians. They also experienced that several of these points had the ability to release old or stagnant energy as well as absorb new, fresh energy. These are "gates"—doorways, allowing the passage of Qi in and out of the body.

To fully absorb energy from trees, we need to activate and use these gates.

Gates for absorbing earth energy

1. Kidney 1, called "Gushing Spring." This point is on the bottom of the foot, between the second and third metatarsal bones, approximately one third of the distance between the base of the second toe and the heel, in a depression formed when the foot is flexed.

2. Pericardium 8, "Place of Toil." This point is located in the center of the palm, between the 2nd and 3rd metacarpal bones, closer to the 3rd metacarpal bone. When a fist is made, the point is where the tip of the middle finger touches the palm.

Gates for absorbing Heaven energy

1. Du 20 "Baihui" or "1000 Meeting Points." This point is located on the top of the head, in a subtle depression above the

tips of the ears, directly above the midpoint of the anterior hairline.

2. Pericardium 8 (see above)

Gates for absorbing energy from nature

1. CV 17, "Sea of Tranquility." This point is located in the center of the sternum in a slight depression, at the level of the fourth intercostal space. On men it lies between the nipples.

2. Pericardium 8 (see above)

FIVE ELEMENT CHART

Element	Metal	Water	Wood	Fire	Earth
Season	Autumn	Winter	Spring	Summer	Late Summer
Color	White	Dark Blue	Green	Red	Yellow
Sound	Sssssss	Choooo	Shhhhh	Haaaaa	Whoooo
Neg. Emotion	Sadness	Fear	Anger	Hatred	Worry
Pos. Emotion	Courage	Tranquillity	Friendliness	Love	Balance
Yin Organ	Lungs	Kidneys	Liver	Heart	Spleen
Yang Organ	Large Intestine	Bladder	Gall Bladder	Small Intestine	Stomach
Sense Organ	Nose	Ears	Eyes	Tongue	Mouth

REFERENCES

1. Davidson, Hilda Roderick Ellis. *Gods and Myths of Northern Europe*, London, and NY, 1990

2. Ronnberg, Ami and Martin, Kathleen. *The Book of Symbols*. Taschen, 2010. P. 128

3. Tolle, Eckhart. *The Power of Now*. New World Press Novato, CA, 1999, P5.

4. Tolle, Eckhart. *Stillness Speaks*. Namaste Publishers, 2003, p. 5

5. Wohlllenben, Peter. *The Hidden Life of Trees*. Graystone Books. Vancouver, BC, Canada 2015.

6. Hanh, Thich Nhat. *Breathe! You are Alive*. Parallax Press, Berkeley, CA, 1996

7. Kirkwood, John. *The Way of the Five Elements*. Singing Dragon, London, UK. 2016.

CPSIA information can be obtained
at www.ICGtesting.com
Printed in the USA
LVHW071337150723
752293LV00006B/266